259/81

Dr Ante Bilić
liječnik - stomatolog

Ante Bilić

19. 03. 81

EXERCISES IN DENTAL RADIOLOGY

VOLUME 2

ADVANCED ORAL RADIOGRAPHIC INTERPRETATION

ROBERT P. LANGLAIS, B.A., D.D.S., M.S.

Associate Professor, and Head of Graduate Program in the
Dental Diagnostic Sciences, Department of Oral Diagnosis
and Roentgenology, University of Texas Health Center at
San Antonio, San Antonio, Texas.

KENNETH C. BENTLEY, D.D.S., M.D., C.M.

Professor, Division of Oral Surgery, Dean, Faculty of
Dentistry, McGill University, Montreal, Canada.

1979

W. B. SAUNDERS COMPANY Philadelphia / London / Toronto

W. B. Saunders Company: West Washington Square
Philadelphia, PA 19105

1 St. Anne's Road
Eastbourne, East Sussex BN21 3UN, England

1 Goldthorne Avenue
Toronto, Ontario M8Z 5T9, Canada

Library of Congress Cataloging in Publication Data

Langlais, Robert P

Advanced oral radiographic interpretation.

(Exercises in dental radiology; v. 2)

1. Teeth — Radiography — Problems, exercises, etc.   2. Teeth
   — Diseases — Diagnosis — Problems, exercises, etc.
   3. Teeth — Diseases — Cases, clinical reports, statistics.
   I. Bentley, Kenneth C., joint author.   II. Title.
   III. Series. [DNLM: 1. Radiography, Dental —
   Examination questions. WN18 L282e 1978]

RK309.L33   617.6'07'572   79–1402
ISBN 0–7216–5616–1

Exercises in Dental Radiology — Volume 2

Advanced Oral Radiographic Interpretation   ISBN 0-7216-5616-1

Last digit is the print number: 9   8   7   6   5   4   3   2   1

*To Professor Emeritus Arthur Gerald Racey, D.D.S.; F.I.C.D.; F.A.C.D.,
our "first teacher" and inspiration for this work.*

FOREWORD

Volume 1 of this series furnished a good review of intra-oral radiographic interpretation. This subject is certainly important because much of dental radiology involves intra-oral radiographs. However, there are many conditions that cannot be interpreted from these radiographs alone. Thus, the subject at hand becomes the basis for *Advanced Oral Radiographic Interpretation.*

Volume 2 differs from Volume 1 because more sophisticated radiographic examinations are shown for the case histories. Various types of extra-oral examinations will require the reader to develop interpretive knowledge above and beyond that required for intra-oral radiography.

Francis Bacon said, "A man is but what he knoweth." This could be paraphrased to mean, "You won't interpret it if you don't know it." Building interpretive acumen is a continuing process—for the student certainly—but also for the general practitioner and for the radiographic specialist. Developing interpretive background is similar to having a bank account. The more money that is placed in the account, the more that can be withdrawn. The more knowledge of radiographic conditions that we store in our brain, the more knowledge we have for making a radiographic interpretation.

The authors' approach to help us learn is an excellent one; they ask us to think. They present the patient's history, combined with the radiograph, and ask us to correlate clinical findings, laboratory data, and radiographic evidence to arrive at a differential diagnosis. This exercise provides us with the opportunity to withdraw interpretive knowledge and also to place new knowledge in the bank.

I hope the reader will avail himself or herself of the opportunity to improve their interpretive skills by avoiding the common tendency to look at the answers too quickly.

Robert E. Silha, D.D.S., M.S.,
F.I.C.D., F.A.A.D.R.

PREFACE

Volume 2 in the series **Exercises in Dental Radiology** is designed to increase the reader's knowledge of roentgenographic interpretation by developing a differential diagnosis, and then, by correlating the remaining pertinent information given, arriving at a final or definitive diagnosis.

We have included 88 actual cases along with the history, the symptoms, and the physical and laboratory findings. Some cases are supported by clinical photographs as well as photomicrographs.

The case histories, along with the pertinent findings and radiographs, were selected because they typify the condition for which a diagnosis is being sought. Remember that information such as age, sex, race, symptoms, laboratory findings, clinical findings, radiographic appearance, and location are all important clues to be used in order to arrive at a diagnosis. Most of the radiographs in this volume are typical of the condition that is being described.

For the convenience of our readers we have used the International Tooth Numbering System. If you are not familiar with this, refer to page 152 for the chart. Each tooth is represented by a two-digit number. The first digit refers to the quadrant. Teeth in the upper right quadrant begin with the number 1; upper left quadrant, number 2; lower left quadrant, number 3; and lower right quadrant, number 4. So, the first number is 1, 2, 3, or 4 and refers to the quadrant. The second number refers to the tooth. The third molar is number 8, the second molar is number 7, the second bicuspid is number 5, and the central incisor is number 1. So, if tooth number 23 is referred to, the first digit represents the quadrant—the upper left, and the second digit represents the tooth—3—which, in this case, is the cuspid. Therefore, number 23 refers to the maxillary left cuspid. Number 47 refers to the mandibular right second molar, and so on. The International Tooth Numbering Code for deciduous teeth has not been included here because no deciduous teeth are referred to by code number in this volume. This has been done to avoid confusion.

As the reader progresses through this volume, he will discover that some conditions are repeated in different cases. This has been done for several reasons: First, some conditions change radiographically through various stages of the disease, and some conditions may have more than one "typical" radiographic appearance. Second, the reader would be placed at a disadvantage if he were able to rule out one or more conditions simply because they had already been presented in a previous case. Therefore, some disease entities have been purposely repeated for the further edification of the reader and to encourage, as much as is possible, objectivity within this unit as a learning experience. It is also for this reason that cases are presented in no particular order or groupings of similar conditions.

We hope that you enjoy this volume, whether it be to reinforce your previous knowledge or to acquire new knowledge in this most challenging aspect of dental radiographic interpretation.

R. P. L.
K. C. B.

ACKNOWLEDGMENTS

We wish to express our sincere thanks to our colleagues who referred these most interesting cases to us. We would also like to thank those fellow dentists who very kindly allowed us to use some of their material. Their names are mentioned under the illustrations that they provided. In particular, we would like to thank Dr. Axel Ruprecht and Dr. Ed Shields for their guidance in diagnosing several of these cases.

We would also like to thank Mr. Haigazoun Artinian and Mr. Joe Donohue for the tremendous effort that they made to provide us with the excellent illustrations seen in this volume. A special note of thanks goes to Mrs. Jill Warzycki, who did an outstanding job of typing the manuscript. We would also like to thank our wives Denyse and Jean, who constantly supported and encouraged us in our efforts to prepare the manuscript.

CONTENTS

CONTENTS

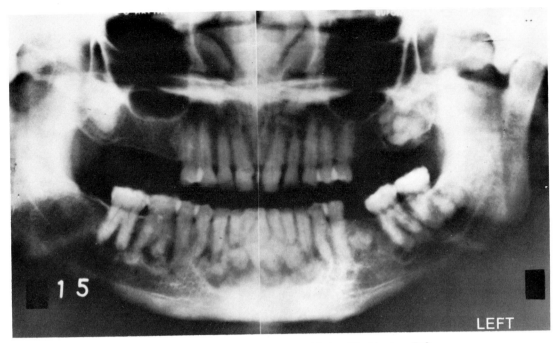

FIGURE 1. Courtesy of Dr. Carson Mader, Washington, D.C.

CASE 1

This 42 year old black female had no symptomatology, and all of her remaining teeth responded positively to the vitalometer pulp test.

On clinical examination, there was no evidence of expansion of the mandible or the maxilla nor were there any areas tender to palpation. No significant periodontal disease was present, and there was no history of trauma or injury to the jaws.

What condition is present?

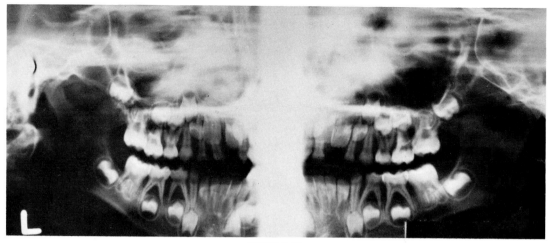

FIGURE 2A

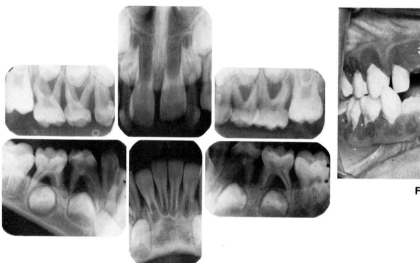

FIGURE 2B

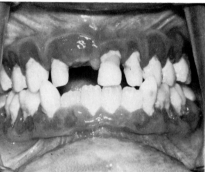

FIGURE 2C

CASE 2

A six year old boy of East Indian origin presents to your office with a complaint of relatively painless swollen gingivae and early loosening of the deciduous teeth. His mother states that the condition began at age three years with bleeding gums and pain when crusty or coarse foods were eaten. The condition persisted, despite the abundance of fresh citrus fruits that she included in his diet. During the previous year, the patient received a complete systemic work-up at the Children's Hospital, from which the following data were obtained:

Hemoglobin (Hgb)	12.0 gm
White blood (cell) count (WBC)	6700
Reticulocyte count	1.2%
Hematocrit (Hct)	37%
Mean corpuscular hemoglobin concentration (MCHC)	32.5%
Urine	Normal
Urine chromatogram (amino acid)	Normal
Calcium	10.4 mg/100 ml
Phosphorus	5.5 mg/100 ml
Alkaline phosphatase	13 King-Armstrong units
Erythrocyte sedimentation rate (ESR)	42 mm/hr
Glucose tolerance	Normal
Fasting blood sugar (glucose) (FBS)	80 mg/100 ml

These tests were repeated on several occasions at timed intervals, and except for the elevated ESR, all were within normal limits for a six year old child. At the time of examination, the patient had taken no medication other than antibiotics and appeared to be a bright, alert, active six year old boy.

Plaque smears and culture and sensitivity tests revealed normal oral flora. These organisms were resistant to penicillin, erythromycin, and tetracycline and were sensitive to clindamycin, ampicillin and cephalexin.

The skeletal survey was normal. There were no findings compatible with hyperparathyroidism or histiocytosis X. There was no calcification in the falx cerebri. The panoramic and intra-oral radiographs (Figs. 2A and 2B) revealed severe, generalized alveolar bone loss about the deciduous teeth.

Gingival biopsy revealed chronic gingivitis with areas of ulceration.

The head and neck examination revealed tender, swollen submaxillary lymph nodes. Intra-orally, the tonsils appeared larger than normal, and a generalized gingival enlargement was noted. In some areas, the surface epithelium appeared desquamated, with a striking, brilliant red color (Fig. 2C). The posterior deciduous teeth were mobile. Note that in the radiographs, alveolar bone loss is minimal about the permanent teeth.

QUESTIONS

1. Give a differential diagnosis.

2. Give a final diagnosis, and substantiate your answer.

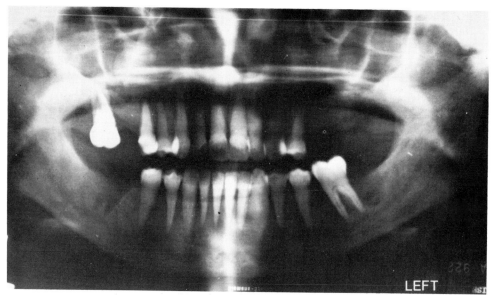

FIGURE 3A. (Taken one year ago)

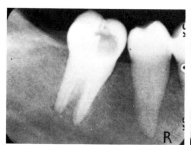

FIGURE 3B.
(Taken one year ago)

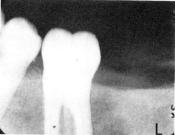

FIGURE 3C.
(Taken one year ago)

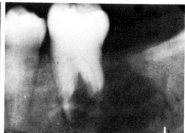

FIGURE 3E.
(Taken at examination)

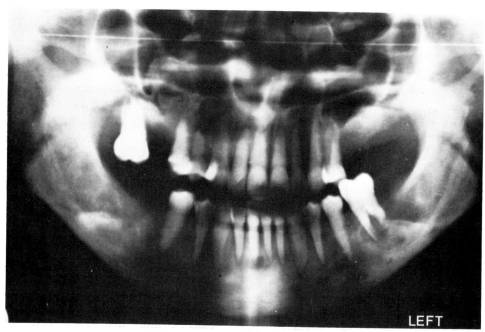

FIGURE 3D. (Taken at examination)
FIGURES 3A–E. Courtesy of Dr. Eric Millar, Montreal, Canada.

CASE 3

Mary Jones is a 26 year old Caucasian female who has been suffering from chronic glomerulonephritis for many years. She has a history of lower back pain, polyuria, and polydipsia and also a history of progressive increases in urea nitrogen (BUN) concentration, as well as increased serum uric acid levels. On testing, the serum calcium level was 12.3 mg/100 ml, the serum inorganic PO_4 level was 1.6 mg/100 ml, and the serum alkaline phosphatase level was 16 King-Armstrong units. Urinary excretion of calcium on a low-calcium diet was 205 mg/liter. There were also elevated levels of urinary hydroxyproline.

The radiograph seen in Figure 3A was taken one year previously. Note the recent extraction socket of the lower right first molar. Figure 3B shows the carious lower right first molar prior to extraction. The periapical radiograph of the lower left first molar was taken at the same time (Fig. 3C). The panoramic radiograph seen in Figure 3D was taken at her most recent visit. The periapical radiograph of the left mandibular first molar was taken at the same time (Fig. 3E). This tooth, though it responded positively to the vitalometer, was extracted, and the radiolucent lesion at its apex was biopsied. The pathologic report confirmed the presence of a central fibrous lesion with giant cells in the left mandible.

QUESTIONS

1. Give a differential diagnosis.

2. Give a substantiated definitive diagnosis.

3. Give a description of the abnormalities as seen in these radiographs.

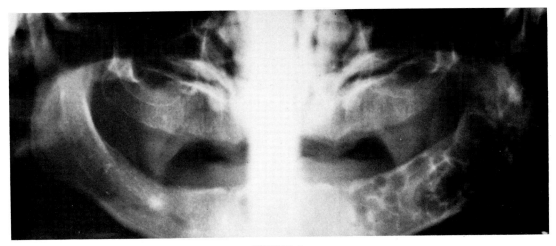

FIGURE 4

CASE 4

Jean François Braconier is a 36 year old man who complained that his lower complete denture no longer fit properly. He had noticed that his occlusion appeared to have changed and that the denture was no longer stable on the lower ridge. Upon examination, the ridge appeared somewhat expanded labially, and a smooth soft-tissue swelling was palpable on one side just buccal to the retromolar pad area. No fluid could be aspirated from the area. He had been edentulous since the age of 16 years but had waited until age 23 years to have the third molars removed. Based upon the biopsy, a hemimandibulectomy was performed. At the time of re-examination, the patient had been free of disease for five years.

QUESTIONS

1. Give a differential diagnosis for the lesion seen in this radiograph.

2. What is your most likely choice?

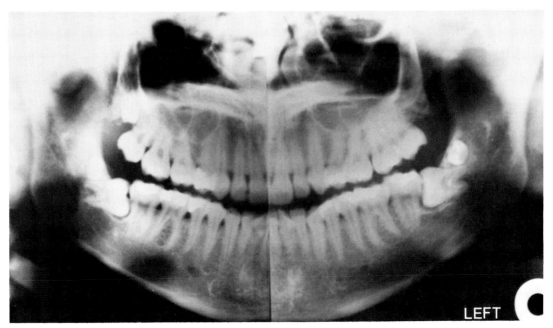

FIGURE 5

CASE 5

This 23 year old Caucasian male presented with pain in the left side of his face. Clinically, the upper left third molar was erupting buccally. He indicated that the pain was most severe in the morning and seemed to diminish during the day.

QUESTIONS

1. What syndrome are these symptoms associated with?

2. Name two syndromes involving supernumerary teeth.

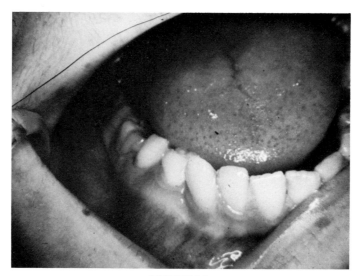

FIGURE 6A

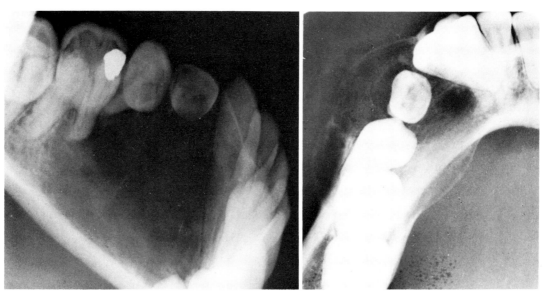

FIGURE 6B   FIGURE 6C

CASE 6

Jim Dandy, a 14 year old Caucasian male, presented with a complaint of swelling of the right lower jaw (Fig. 6A). The patient had noticed a small lump in the right mental region one year previously. The mass has slowly increased in size since that time. The lesion is asymptomatic, and there is no loss of sensation of the lower lip. There are no skin lesions, and there has been no loss of weight.

The Hgb, Hct, WBC, and differential are all within normal limits. The calcium and phosphorus levels are normal, and the alkaline phosphatase level is 27.8 King-Armstrong units. (The normal value for this age group is <25 King-Armstrong units.) The skeletal survey is within normal limits.

QUESTIONS

1. Before proceeding further, give a differential diagnosis for the lesion, keeping in mind the patient's age, the radiographic appearance, and the location of the lesion.

2. After you have made your differential diagnosis, it is learned that the pathology report described a lesion characterized by a dense, fibrous connective tissue stroma interspersed with islands of normal lamellar bone. What is your final impression?

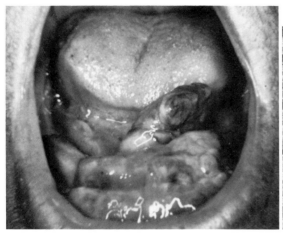

FIGURE 7A

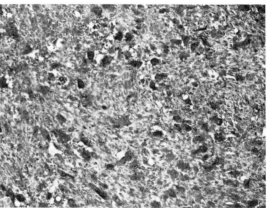

FIGURE 7B

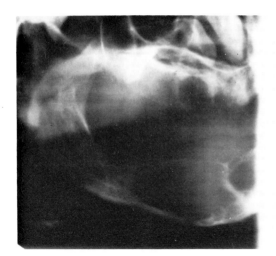

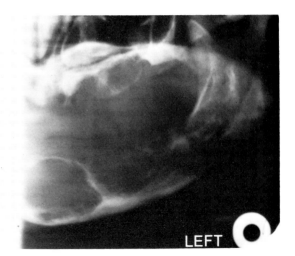

FIGURE 7C

CASE 7

Mrs. Montrealopoulos, a 34 year old female of Greek origin, presented with a complaint of being unable to wear her lower denture. Six months earlier she had observed a small, purplish-red mass near the lingual flange of her lower denture at the midline. The mass had grown progressively larger and bled easily when touched. She had no pain and no history of trauma. She revealed that she had a similar small lesion removed from the right maxillary gingiva three years before.

The laboratory data consisted of the following:

Hgb	8.5 gm
Hct	30%
WBC	6600, normal differential
Calcium	11.2 mg/100 ml (normal 9–11 mg/100 ml)
Phosphorus	2.0 mg/100 ml (normal 2.5–4.5 mg/100 ml)
Alkaline phosphatase	8.5 King-Armstrong units (normal 3–13 King-Armstrong units)
BUN	10 mg/100 ml (normal 10–20 mg/100 ml)
24-hour urinary calcium	84.5 mg/liter (normal 150 mg/liter)
Intravenous pyelogram (IVP)	Within normal limits
Tubular reabsorption of phosphate	Within normal limits
Biopsy	See Fig. 7B.
Skeletal survey	Within normal limits
Blood smear	Hypochromic, microcytic anemia
Reticulocyte count	6.4%

Using the data given and the illustrations, give your diagnosis.

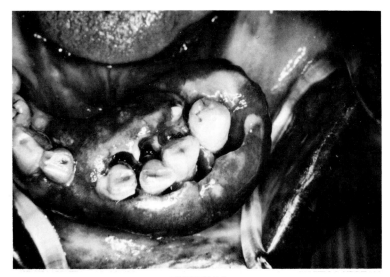

FIGURE 8A

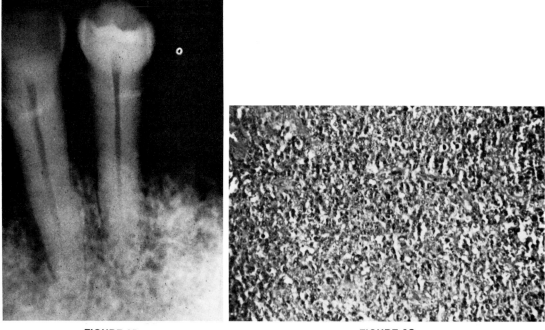

FIGURE 8B   **FIGURE 8C**

FIGURE 8, A–C.   Courtesy of Dr. Eric Millar, Montreal, Canada.

CASE 8

This 80 year old black male of Jamaican origin presented with a complaint of looseness of the lower front teeth. The patient noticed this looseness two months previously, and two weeks later a rapidly growing, purplish-red, friable mass developed around the teeth. At examination, the teeth were painful. Microscopically, the subepithelial connective tissue was filled with sheets of round, large, deeply basophilic cells as well as numerous large multinucleated cells with pale cytoplasms. There were numerous mitotic figures. The area seen in Figure 8C is the lamina propria of the gingiva.

QUESTIONS

Based on the *clinical* findings:

1. What is your differential diagnosis?

2. In visualizing this low-power view of the biopsy specimen (Fig. 8C), what is the most likely choice?

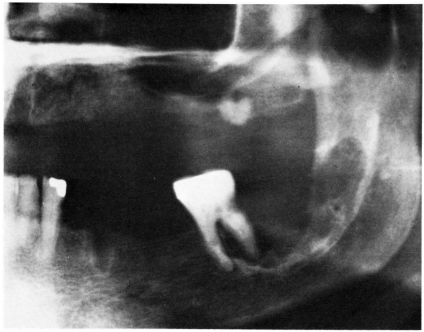

FIGURE 9   **LEFT**

Courtesy of Dr. Paul Luxford, Calgary, Canada.

CASE 9

This Caucasian male patient, aged 74 years, presented with a complaint of pain and swelling in the left lower jaw. The patient had had recurrent pain and swelling over the mandibular third molar area for several months and had noticed loosening of the second molar. The oral mucosa in the area appeared normal. The medical history was unremarkable except for increasing difficulty on urination. Upon aspiration of the mass, a clear mucoid fluid was obtained.

QUESTION

1. Give a differential diagnosis.

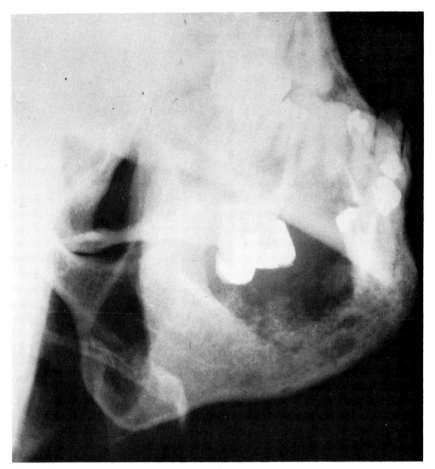

RIGHT   FIGURE 10

CASE 10

This 48 year old Caucasian male had a history of squamous cell carcinoma of the mandibular right posterior gingiva that had been treated with 6200 rads of cobalt 60 over a period of 31 visits. Early in the course of therapy, teeth numbers 35, 36, and 37 were extracted. One year after therapy, the tissue, though slightly thin, appeared normal. A partial lower denture was constructed, and the patient remained asymptomatic for another three years. The patient then developed a periodontitis about most of his remaining teeth, and the partial denture began to rock when he masticated food. This radiograph was taken shortly after the patient presented complaining of pain under his partial denture. Clinically, the alveolar mucosa appeared erythematous, and there were several areas of denuded bone.

QUESTIONS

1. What is your diagnosis?

2. How did this condition develop?

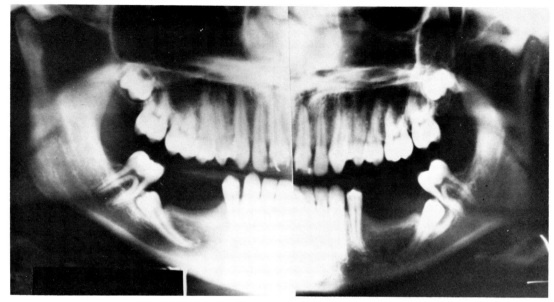

FIGURE 11   **LEFT**

CASE 11

Provide a radiologic report for this radiograph of a 16 year old
Caucasian male patient.

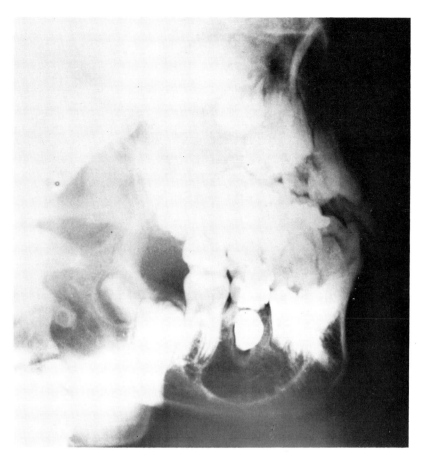

RIGHT   **FIGURE 12**

CASE 12

    1. How old is this patient?

    2. In which direction does tooth number 35 appear to be erupting?

    3. What pathologic findings would you report?

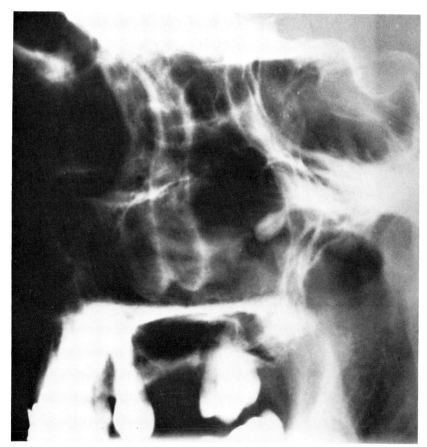

FIGURE 13

CASE 13

What finding(s) would you report after examining this lateral view of the right and left maxillary sinuses?

QUESTIONS

1. Give a differential diagnosis.
2. What is the most likely choice?

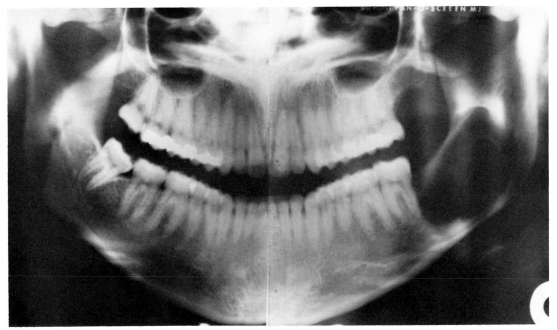

FIGURE 14   LEFT

CASE 14

What is your interpretation of the radiolucency seen on the left side of this patient's mandible. The impacted left third molars were removed five years ago, and the patient is now 25 years of age. There were no complications associated with the surgery. The patient is asymptomatic.

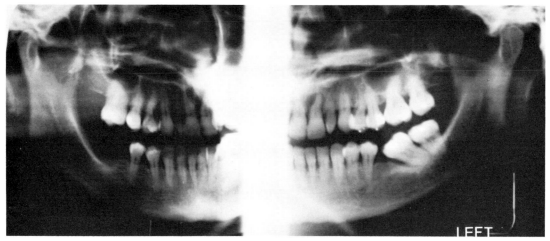

FIGURE 15A

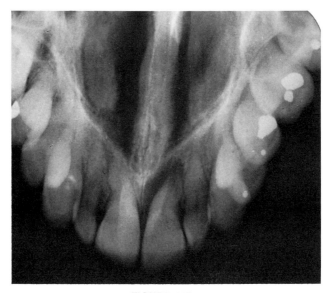

FIGURE 15B

CASE 15

This 56 year old Caucasian female presented with moderate pain in the maxillary anterior region. On examination, one of the maxillary teeth was found to be mobile, and there was a heavy wear facet on the lingual surface.

QUESTIONS

1. Which tooth is involved?

2. What treatment would you suggest?

3. What congenital anomaly is present?

4. Which mandibular tooth has the poorest prognosis? Why?

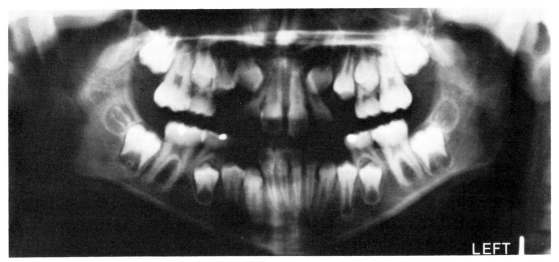

FIGURE 16A. Courtesy of Dr. Eddie Slapcoff, Montreal, Canada.

CASE 16

This 10 year old Caucasian female is under the care of an orthodontist. Serial extractions have been performed. The orthodontist has not been contemplating the extraction of any permanent teeth, but based on this radiograph, he is now considering the possibility of extracting a permanent tooth. The patient is asymptomatic.

QUESTIONS

    1. Which tooth will be extracted?

    2. Why?

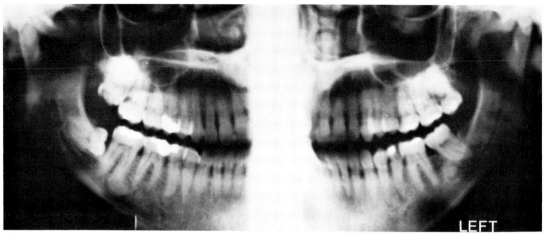

FIGURE 17
Courtesy of Dr. A. Namin, Montreal, Canada.

CASE 17

This patient is a 45 year old black female. She has pain in the right posterior mandibular area. There is a history of trismus that cleared up after antibiotic therapy.

QUESTIONS

1. What treatment would you prescribe?

2. Give a differential diagnosis for the radiopaque lesion associated with the apex of the mandibular right second molar.

3. In viewing the radiograph, list as many other pathologic processes as possible.

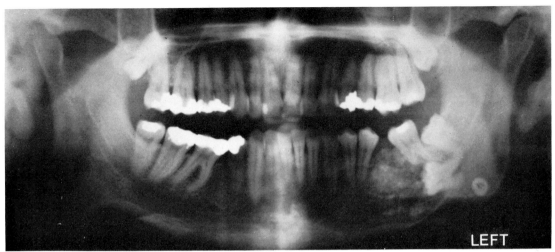

FIGURE 18A. Courtesy of Dr. M. Gornitsky, Montreal, Canada.

CASE 18

This 32 year old Caucasian male patient presented with mild paresthesia in the lower lip on the left side. He stated that he knew he had four impacted teeth and that this was probably the cause.

Intra-orally, there was no evidence of expansion of the left mandibular cortical plates, and the overlying soft tissue appeared healthy. There were no detectable fistulae at the time of examination.

QUESTIONS

1. Give a differential diagnosis for the lesion seen in this radiograph.

2. With the aid of the photomicrographs in the answer section, give your diagnosis.

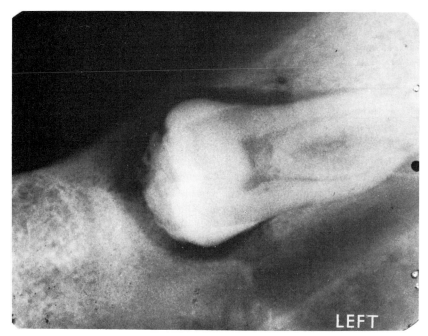

FIGURE 19*A*

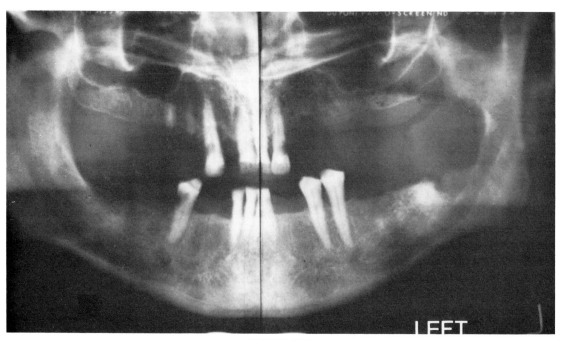

FIGURE 19*B*

CASE 19

This 74 year old Caucasian male, who was in no acute distress, presented with an area of drainage in the mandibular left third molar region. He was in apparent good health and was taking no specific medications. He was wearing partial upper and lower dentures and stated that he had recently developed a little soreness under the lower partial denture on the left side. The periapical radiograph (Fig. 19A) revealed a horizontally impacted lower left third molar with a 2-mm radiolucent area surrounding the crown of the tooth and an additional tract-like area leading to the mandibular canal. The impression was that this was an "infected impaction," and the tooth was removed. No pathologic examination was carried out.

Over the next nine months, the patient had persistent pain and swelling at the extraction site. Antibiotics were prescribed several times, each time the area was curetted and packed with medicated gauze; and each time the patient initially improved but eventually returned in distress. The patient ultimately developed swelling and tenderness on the left side of the face as well as a firm, swollen area in the left retromolar pad area. There was no paresthesia of the lip. At this time, radiograph 19B was taken, and the area was biopsied.

What is your impression?

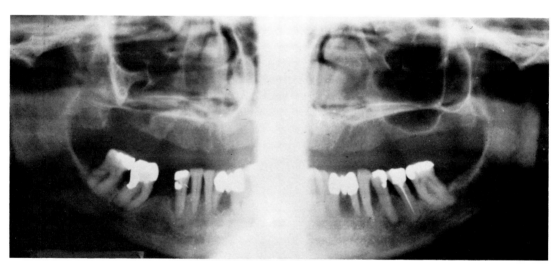

FIGURE 20

CASE 20

This 70 year old white female, actively employed as the manager of a prestigious private social club, was referred for a consultation because she had recently begun to have gingival bleeding and mild discomfort in her mandibular teeth. She had been treated with antibiotics and gingival curettage at one-month intervals for the past three months, but the problem persisted.

Although she appeared healthy, she was being treated with diuretics for mild hypertension, and over the past year she had lost 20 pounds. She complained of drowsiness and a lack of strength, especially toward midafternoon. She had recently taken to "snacking," and although she enjoyed this, she wondered why she was not gaining weight. She claimed that she always drank large quantities of tea at work and at home and usually got up several times during the night to urinate. She stated that she had recently been treated for a mycotic vaginitis and that she had been troubled with kidney and bladder infections for many years.

The routine hemogram was normal, including indices. There was a slightly elevated ESR and a WBC of 12,500. The BUN was 15 mg/100 ml (normal is 8–18 mg/100 ml), and the 12-hour FBS was 114 mg/100 ml (normal is 60–100 mg/100 ml). The urinary glucose level was high normal. The glucose tolerance test revealed a one-hour serum glucose of 220 mg/100 ml and a three-hour serum glucose of 180 mg/100 ml.

What is your impression?

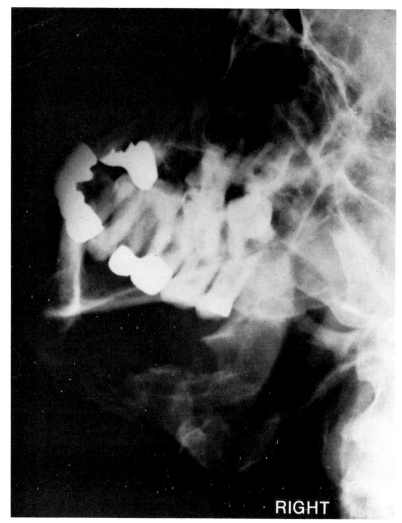

FIGURE 21

CASE 21

This 47 year old Caucasian male patient first presented eight months ago for removal of a retained root tip in the mandibular right molar area. The patient was edentulous in the mandible and had noticed that his lower denture was no longer comfortable. The root tip was removed in a routine procedure.

The socket failed to heal, however, and the patient developed acute pain at the extraction site. He was then seen on a weekly basis over a seven-week period. Dressings were placed in the socket, and two five-day courses of penicillin V were administered. The patient improved and was not seen for another three months. Approximately five months after the original extraction, the patient returned still complaining that he could not wear his mandibular denture. Radiographically, the body of the mandible revealed a "moth-eaten" appearance and a large segment of bone along with some five smaller segments could be seen to be separated from the body of the mandible just beneath the epithelium. Several drainage fistulae were present, and the soft tissue overlying the ridge was red and slightly edematous. The patient's oral temperature was 99.5°F. The routine hemogram was normal except for a WBC of 13,700. The gallium scan of the right mandible showed a large "hot" area in the mandibular molar-bicuspid area. A sequestrectomy was performed, and the patient was placed on long-term antibiotic therapy. Culture and sensitivity tests revealed the organisms to be penicillin resistant.

QUESTIONS

1. What is your impression?

2. What treatment would you recommend?

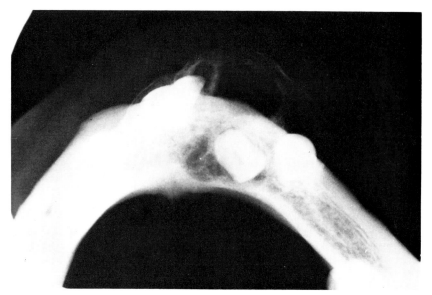

FIGURE 22A

CASE 22

This 42 year old French Canadian hockey player received a blow to the anterior region of the mandible. A day later he felt a "lump" on his chin and was referred to the club dentist. This radiograph was taken at the time of examination. The periapical view revealed a vertically impacted, unerupted mandibular cuspid tooth and an altered trabecular pattern in the region. The biopsy specimen is seen in the answer section.

Give your diagnosis.

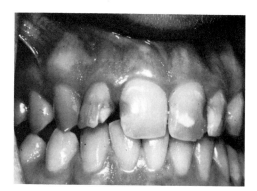

FIGURE 23A

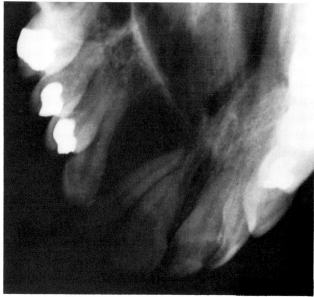

RIGHT   FIGURE 23B

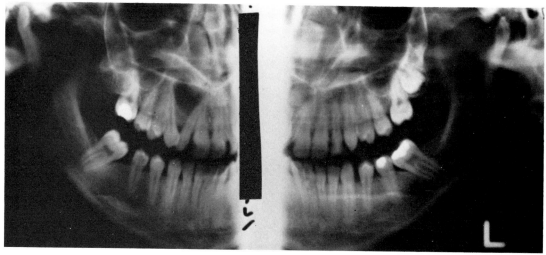

FIGURE 23C

32

CASE 23

This 23 year old white female presented to the hospital emergency clinic with mild discomfort in the maxillary anterior area. She also complained that her right lateral incisor had been getting progressively darker in color, and it also seemed to be more "crooked" than before. There was no history of trauma, and on examination, the tooth had large mesial and distal restorations. The tooth was not sensitive to percussion, hot, or cold and did not respond to the electric pulp test. A parulis was noted in the apical region between teeth numbers 12 and 13.

QUESTIONS

1. Give a differential diagnosis.
2. What treatment would you prescribe? Be complete.

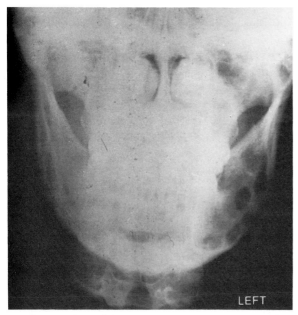

FIGURE 24A

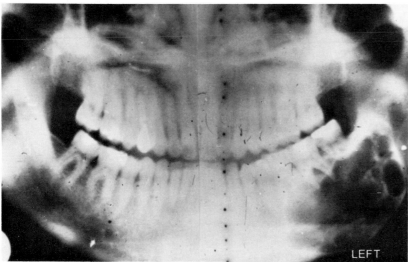

FIGURE 24B

CASE 24

This 34 year old Japanese male patient was seen with a complaint of deep, constant pain of two days' duration in the lower left molar area. The clinical examination revealed expansion of the body of the mandible laterally, medially, and inferiorly. Slight swelling and lymphadenopathy were present in the left submandibular area. The first, second, and third molars were sensitive to percussion. The intra-oral periapical view revealed a deep carious lesion of the third molar. The laboratory work-up consisted of Hct, Hgb, WBC and differential, BUN, serum calcium, PO_4, and alkaline phosphatase levels. All were within normal limits.

Surgically, thin gelatinous globular masses, which easily separated from the bone leaving a smooth, shiny surface, were removed. The biopsy report described tissue resembling the normal dental papilla. The area healed but was observed closely, as recurrence was thought to be possible.

What is your impression? Note the photomicrograph of the lesion in the answer section (Fig. 24C).

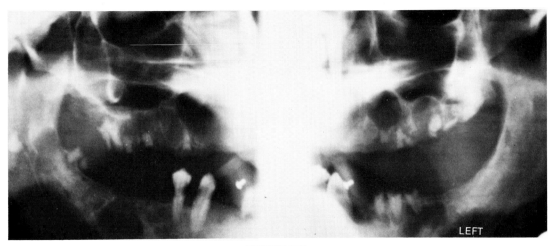

FIGURE 25A

CASE 25

This 64 year old Caucasian male presented to the emergency dental clinic with mild discomfort and pain in his mouth. He was visibly apprehensive and stated that he "hated" dentists but that he was tired of having constant discomfort in his mouth. He was planning to retire soon, and he felt that he "owed" himself a decent set of teeth, the purchase of which was something he had meant to do for years.

The two-month postoperative radiograph can be seen in the answer section (Fig. 25B).

What is your impression?

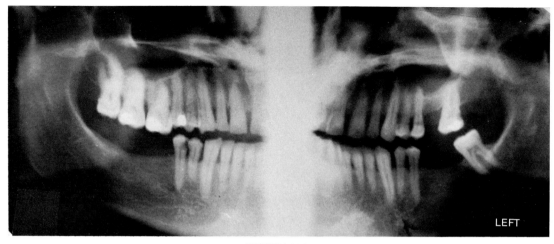

FIGURE 26A

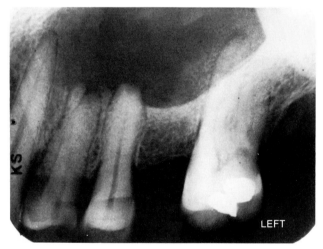

FIGURE 26B

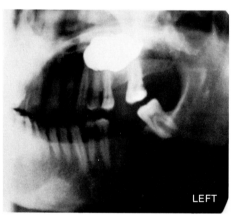

FIGURE 26C

CASE 26

This 45 year old Caucasian male presented with a tender, fluctuant swelling in the upper left mucobuccal fold of four or five weeks' duration. Pain was aggravated by bending over or rapidly descending a staircase. The upper right second bicuspid showed marked gingival recession on the buccal aspect as well as severe toothbrush abrasion and proved to be nonreactive to hot, cold, and electric pulp tests. The panoramic and periapical radiographs can be seen in Figures 26*A* and 26*B*. The left maxillary sinus did not transilluminate and was tender to palpation in the infra-orbital area. A 19-gauge needle was inserted into the fluctuant area, and 5 ml of brownish, somewhat mucoid fluid were drawn off. Five ml of radiopaque medium were injected into the area, and radiograph 26*C* was taken. Gentle blowing through the occluded nose revealed no communication between the oral and nasal cavities. A layer of tissue was peeled away from the wall of the cavity, and healing eventually took place. Root canal therapy was performed on the upper left second bicuspid, periodontal therapy was instituted, and the patient remained asymptomatic.

What is your impression?

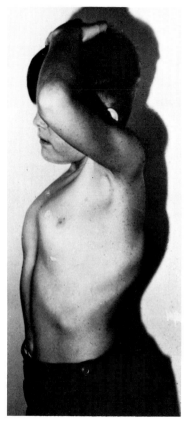

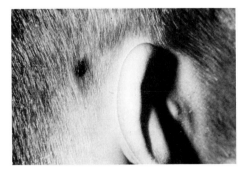

FIGURE 27B

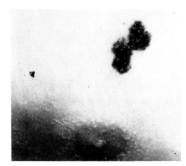

FIGURE 27A **FIGURE 27C**

FIGURE 27, *A–F.* Courtesy of Dr. Simon Weinberg, Toronto, Canada.

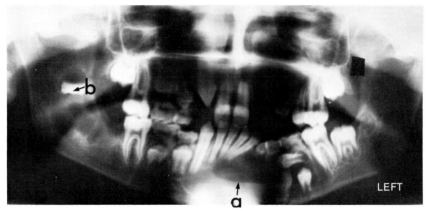

FIGURE 27D

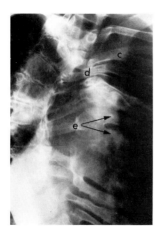

FIGURE 27E

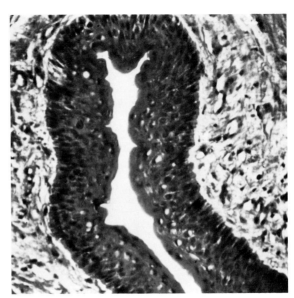

FIGURE 27F

CASE 27

The findings seen in this case are typical of this condition. What condition affects this 12 year old boy?

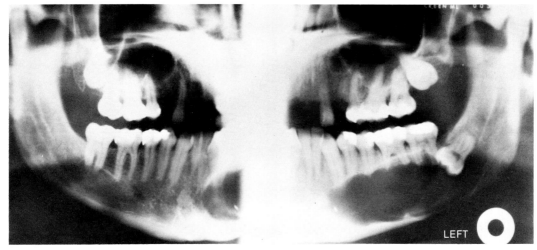
FIGURE 28

CASE 28

Identify, as specifically as you can, the large radiolucent area located in the body of the left mandible of this 23 year old asymptomatic Caucasian male.

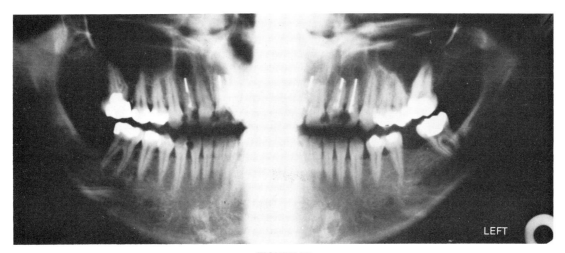

FIGURE 29

CASE 29

Six months ago, this 35 year old Caucasian female patient had three apicoectomies in the anterior area. Previous to this, there had been a one-year history of chronic "blow-ups" of the endodontically treated teeth.

What is your impression of the radiolucent area of the apex of the right maxillary lateral incisor?

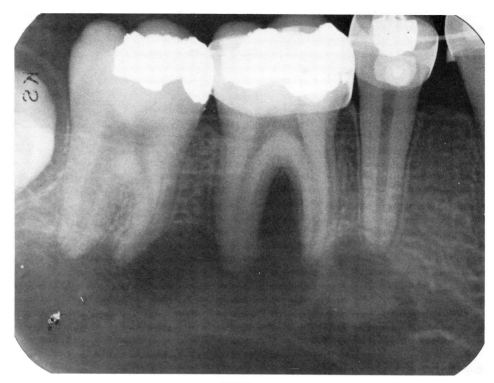

FIGURE 30

CASE 30

This 14 year old female patient, who was undergoing orthodontic treatment, was discovered to have a large radiolucent area, which developed sometime after treatment was started one year ago. She was completely asymptomatic, and no history of trauma could be elicited. There was no evidence of expansion clinically.

The area was explored surgically, and an empty cavity was found. Subsequently, the area healed within 14 months.

QUESTION

1. What is your diagnosis?

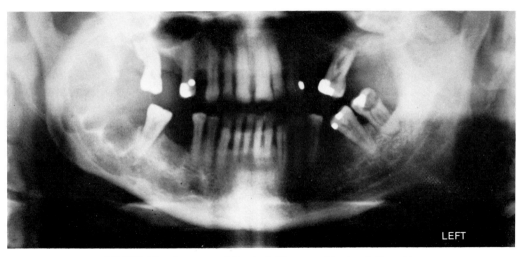

FIGURE 31. Courtesy of Dr. Jack Sherman, Montreal, Canada.

CASE 31

This 44 year old Caucasian patient was in for a routine check-up when the family dentist discovered a firm but yielding swelling just buccal to the third molar area in the right mandible. The overlying mucosa appeared intact. The area was asymptomatic. The patient was in good systemic health and had no dermatologic conditions.

At surgery, a cavity was found that was filled with a straw-colored fluid intermixed with some white "curdy" material.

With this information, what is your impression?

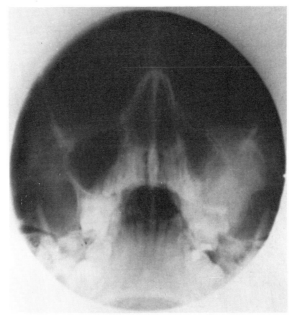

FIGURE 32A   LEFT

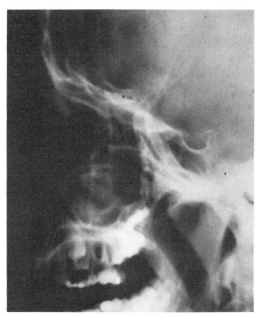

FIGURE 32B

CASE 32

This 10 year old patient presented with swelling of the left maxilla, expanding both buccally and into the maxillary sinus. There were no other involved areas, and all laboratory values were normal except for a slightly elevated serum alkaline phosphatase level. The hand films showed no evidence of subperiosteal erosion in the phalanges.

What is your impression?

44

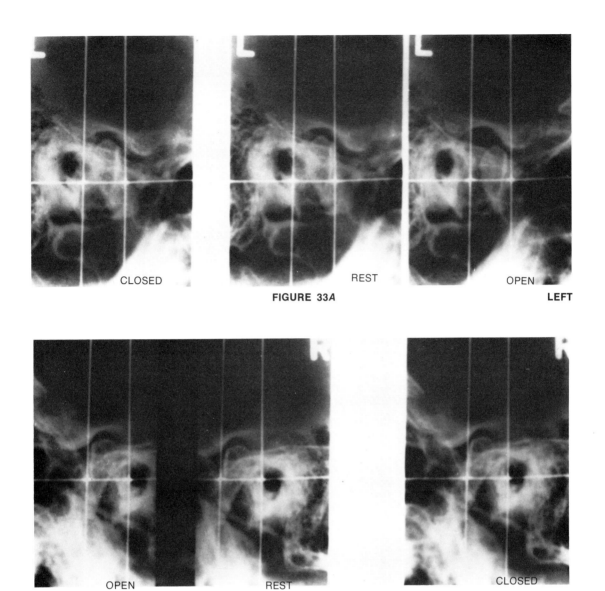

CLOSED

REST

OPEN

FIGURE 33A

LEFT

OPEN

REST

CLOSED

FIGURE 33B

RIGHT

CASE 33

This 34 year old Caucasian female complained of pain in the *left* temporomandibular joint (TMJ) — especially upon opening of the mouth. She also stated that she had severe, frequent unilateral head-aches in the left temporal area, which were sometimes associated with pain over the left side of the face and neck. The severity of the pain was greatest upon arising from bed in the morning. There was marked crepitus and clicking in the *left* TMJ, but this was not always present. She recalled that this pain had begun as a dull, intermittent ache some five years before, but for the past two years she had been actively seeking treatment with no results.

Upon further questioning, she revealed that she had developed psoriasis 18 months earlier. There was no family history of psoriasis and at the time of examination, she had hairline involvement only. History revealed a hysterectomy 10 years before for dysmenorrhea. She also indicated that there was a coexisting lower back problem, which was apparently due to a herniated disc. She was allergic to morphine derivatives and penicillin. Previous treatment consisted of nonnarcotic analgesics, tranquilizers, and intracapsular injections of steroids, the latter providing dramatic but only temporary relief.

The social history revealed that in a fit of rage, her husband had struck her on the *left* side of the face five years earlier. Her husband is a heavy drinker, but she remains happy with her marriage. Until one month ago, she had been a cashier at a local chain food store, but because of the severity of her facial pain, she had passed out several times at her cash register and was now on sick leave.

The physical examination of the head and neck area revealed no palpable lymph nodes or enlargement in the thyroid area, and the soft tissue of the oral cavity appeared normal. Further examination, however, revealed the following:

Palpation of the *left* posterior TMJ, through the external auditory meatus, revealed tenderness; the remaining aspects of both TM joints were normal. The *left* internal (medial) pterygoid muscle and the *left* external (lateral) pterygoid muscle were extremely tender to palpation. At maximum opening of the mandible, the space between the upper and lower teeth was 12 mm; at maximum opening, the midline of the mandible deviated 5 mm to the *right*. There were heavy wear facets on the teeth, and when questioned she stated that her husband had complained many times of the grinding noises she made in her sleep. Finally, she stated that she had spontaneously dislocated her jaw eight months earlier and had to have it "put back" by her physician.

Based on careful consideration of these findings and upon this patient's radiographs, try to answer the following questions.

You will find a duplicate set of radiographs in the answer section.

QUESTIONS

1. What condition(s) or disease(s) is this patient suffering from?

2. Using the radiographs, answer the following:
   a). Describe the *pathologic* changes (if any) in the joints.
   b). Describe the radiographic evidence (if any) of the deviation to the *right*.

3. What finding in the physical examination relates to the clicking in the *left* TMJ?

4. How would you treat this patient?

5. Relative to the history and physical findings, what factors would you use to monitor progress during treatment?

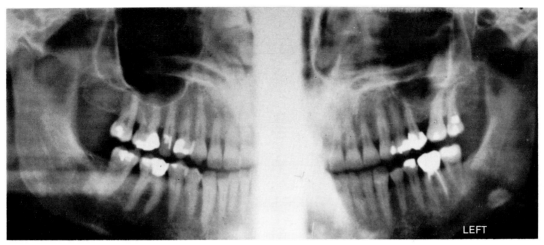

FIGURE 34A. Courtesy of Dr. Ronald Jones, Montreal, Canada.

CASE 34

This patient presented with a history of swelling and discomfort of the left floor of the mouth and submandibular areas.

The condition had improved after antibiotic therapy but continued to recur. The patient was referred for further evaluation and to rule out the possibility of incomplete endodontic therapy as a cause.

What is your impression? (Once you have considered the facts given, you may consult the radiographs in the answer section.)

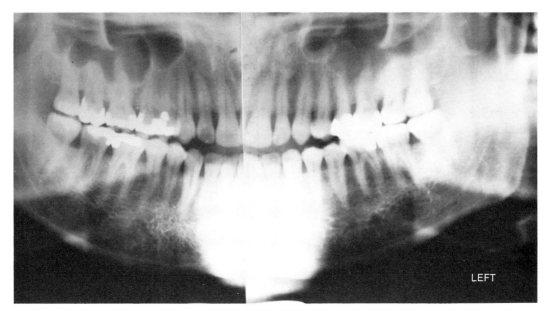

FIGURE 35

CASE 35

This 35 year old female has a complaint of toothache that seems to be located in her right maxillary second molar. Lately, she feels that all of her right maxillary posterior teeth are sore, and at times the left side aches also. The pain is of three weeks' duration and is most acute during the day but is not particularly associated with meals or any specific type of food. She states that when she goes down the stairs at her office or when she is jogging, she becomes acutely aware of her aching teeth.

The clinical examination revealed that all the maxillary teeth responded positively to the vitalometer and that the right maxillary molars and the second bicuspid were sensitive to percussion. The left maxillary first molar was slightly sensitive to percussion. There was no detectable caries, and the gingiva and periodontium appeared to be in excellent condition. She had an occlusal equilibration six months ago, and there did not appear to be any premature contacts.

QUESTIONS

1. What further questions would you ask?
2. What further examination would you carry out?
3. What is your impression?
4. How would you treat this condition?

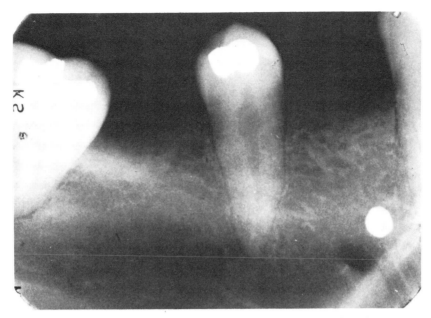

FIGURE 36A. Courtesy of Dr. Elliot Goldberg, Montreal, Canada.

CASE 36

Apart from using the "buccal object rule" (Clark's rule), what simple radiograph may be taken in order to locate this shotgun pellet's position within the lower jaw — buccal or lingual to the mandible.

This view is illustrated in the answer section.

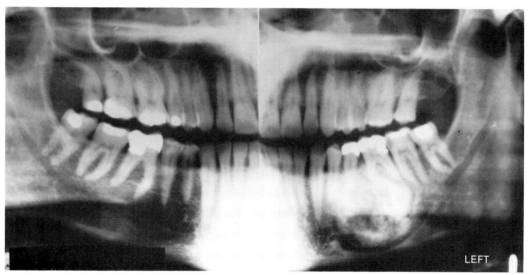

FIGURE 37. Courtesy of Dr. Gary Freedman, Montreal, Canada.

CASE 37

This 34 year old Caucasian male was seen at the time of his routine dental check-up. He complained of intermittent sensitivity to hot and cold in the mandibular left molar region. The large restorations in the area have been present for many years.

His family dentist noted a slight expansion of the buccal and lingual cortical plates in the lower left bicuspid-molar area. None of the teeth were sensitive to percussion and all responded positively to heat, cold, and electric pulp tests. The area was not tender to palpation, and the overlying mucosa appeared normal.

QUESTIONS

1. What is the cause of this patient's symptoms?

2. Give a differential diagnosis for the large radiopaque lesion.

3. What is your best choice?

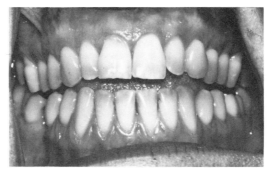

FIGURE 38A. Courtesy of Dr. Nasser Dibai and Dr. Avrum Sonin, Montreal, Canada.

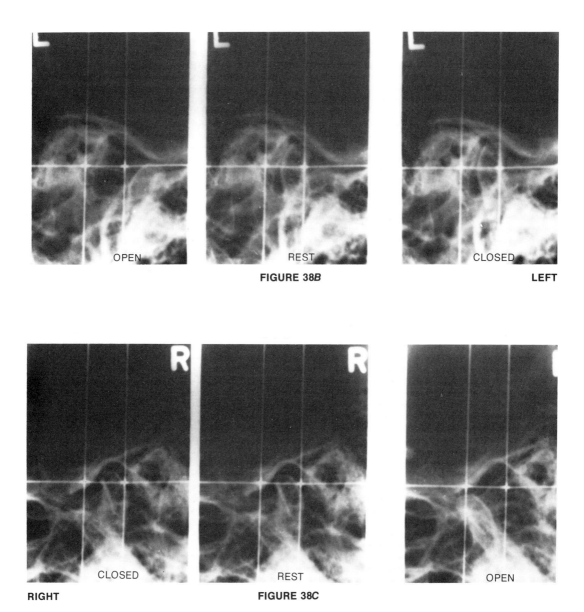

OPEN REST CLOSED

FIGURE 38B LEFT

RIGHT CLOSED REST OPEN

FIGURE 38C

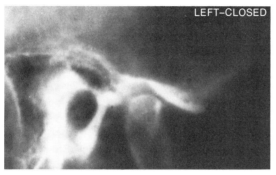

LEFT-CLOSED

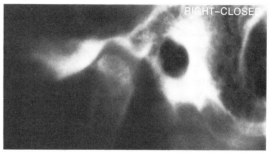

RIGHT-CLOSED

FIGURE 38*D*   FIGURE 38*E*

CASE 38

This 30 year old Caucasian female complained that her jaw felt "lopsided" and that there was pain in the *right* and *left* temporomandibular joints (TMJ). She also said that her teeth no longer came together (Fig. 38*A*). This all began 18 months ago, following a lengthy dental appointment when root canal treatment was completed.

Upon further questioning, she stated that she had crepitus in both joints and that sometimes the pain appeared to be most severe upon awakening in the morning but that at times she would notice it when she was concentrating, such as when she was driving her car. She also stated that she would sometimes awaken during the night with a severe headache in both temporal areas.

Her medical history was unremarkable except for one acute episode of Chinese restaurant syndrome (CRS), which is caused by excessive intake of monosodium glutamate. She described herself as "hyper" by nature and seemed happy with her marriage and her job as a teacher.

The physical examination revealed no tenderness to palpation of either TMJ. There was intense tenderness to palpation of the *right* internal and external pterygoid muscles as well as of the *left* internal and external pterygoid and masseter muscles. Her maximum mouth opening was limited to 35 mm and was painful; there was no deviation. She did, however, protrude her jaw or "translate" extensively upon opening of the mouth. Further questioning established that she was a "bruxer" by night and a "clencher" by day.

The only previous treatment that she had had for this condition was an occlusal adjustment, which proved unsuccessful.

QUESTIONS

1. What radiographic findings (if any) are present?

2. What is your diagnosis?

3. What treatment would you suggest?

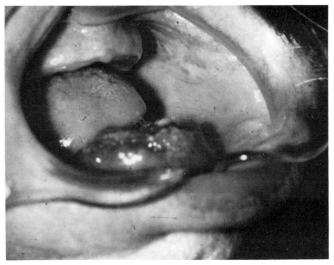

FIGURE 39A

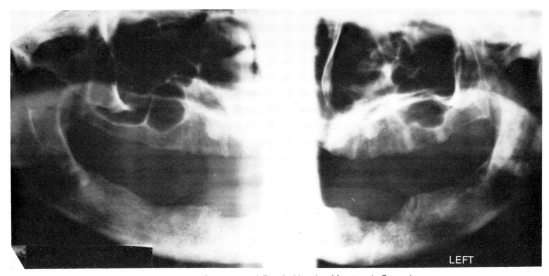

FIGURE 39B. Courtesy of Dr. A. Namin, Montreal, Canada.

CASE 39

This 60 year old Caucasian female complained that she had not been able to wear her lower denture for the past three months and that she had been having trouble with her appliance for three months prior to that.

The physical examination revealed a large, fleshy, indurated mass on the anterior gingiva. There were no palpable lymph nodes of the head and neck region.

QUESTIONS

1. Give a differential diagnosis for this lesion.

2. What is your most likely choice?

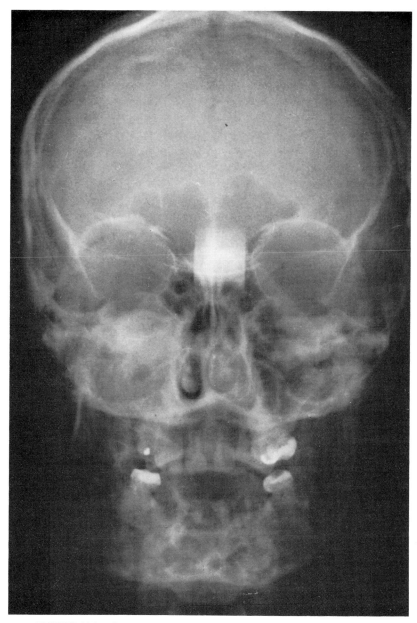

FIGURE 40A. Courtesy of Dr. Ralph MacDonald, Indianapolis, Indiana.

CASE 40

What condition are these radiographs pathognomonic of in this 12 year old female?

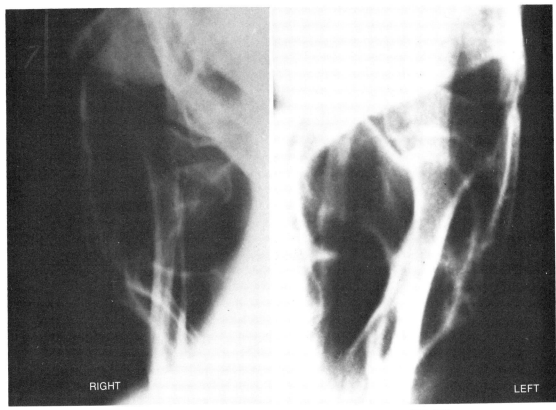

RIGHT

LEFT

FIGURE 41A   **FIGURE 41B**

CASE 41

This patient presented with facial asymmetry, the left side of the face appearing longer than the right side, especially in the lower third.

The patient had no symptoms, and during her history it was discovered that she had been in an automobile accident eight years before.

What is the cause of the facial asymmetry?

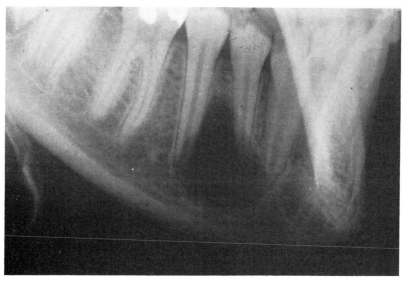

FIGURE 42

CASE 42

This 12 year old girl remembers receiving a blow to the face about one year previously.

The area was explored surgically. An empty cavity was found, and the radiolucency disappeared within eight months.

What is your impression? Be careful, you have seen this before!

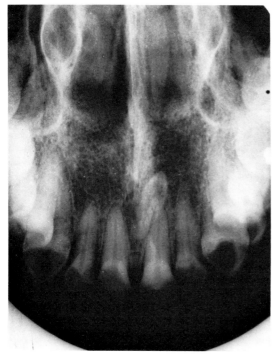

FIGURE 43A

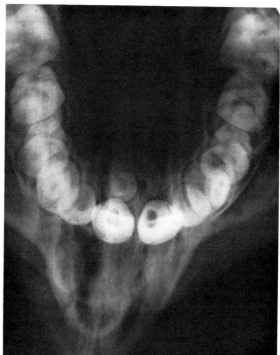

FIGURE 43B

CASE 43

Figure 43A and Figure 43B represent two different patients with the same condition.

QUESTIONS

1. What is the condition?

2. Name the type of radiographic view seen in Figure 43A and Figure 43B.

3. What are the advantages and disadvantages of each?

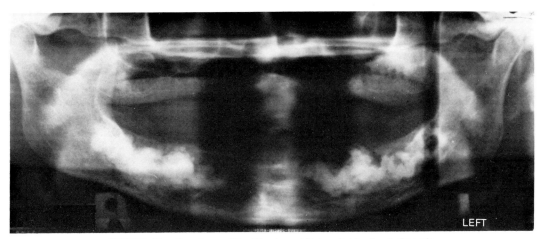

FIGURE 44. Courtesy of Dr. Monique Michaud, Montreal, Canada.

CASE 44

This is a 44 year old black female who is complaining of slight soreness under the left side of the mandibular denture. She had her teeth extracted three years previously because of severe periodontal disease and had been getting along well with her dentures until now.

Clinically, a small fistula was noted in the mandibular left cuspid-bicuspid area. Otherwise, the mouth appeared normal.

QUESTIONS

1. Give a differential diagnosis.
2. What is your best choice?

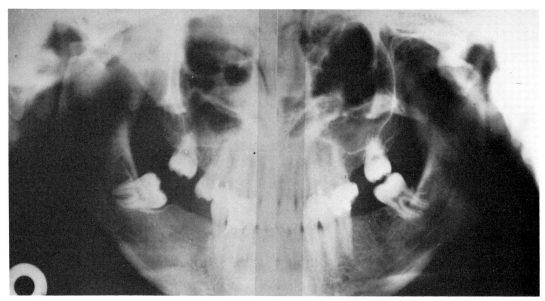

FIGURE 45

CASE 45

John Drinkmore, a 22 year old college student, had been out with the boys one evening and awakened the next morning experiencing extreme discomfort in the preauricular region on both sides. He was unable to chew his breakfast and noticed that his maxillary and mandibular teeth were only making contact in the second and third molar regions. Upward pressure exerted by his hand against his chin, however, would allow the teeth to make contact in the anterior region. The patient did not recall sustaining any trauma, but his friends subsequently informed him that he had been drinking rather heavily that night.

After examining the radiograph, what is your diagnosis?

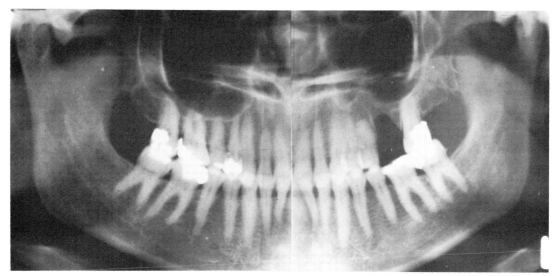

FIGURE 46   LEFT

CASE 46

This 52 year old female was discovered to be a diabetic two years ago. Initially, she was treated for her disease with insulin, and it was subsequently controlled by diet and a long-acting oral hypoglycemic agent. Six months ago she underwent a difficult surgical removal of the left maxillary first molar after which her dentist prescribed antibiotics and instructed her not to blow her nose for 48 hours. Since then she has been aware of a salty taste in the area of the extraction and of a tendency for some fluid to escape from her left nostril when she is drinking fluids.

QUESTIONS

1. What do you think the problem is?

2. How would the problem be managed?

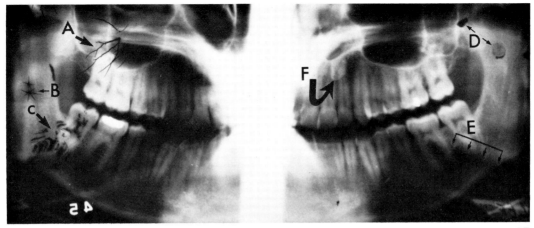

FIGURE 47 LEFT

CASE 47

This case is included just to give you a break and to see if you can pick up a few artifacts.

Identify the causes of the following. (See arrows.)

A. Lightning effect.

B. Starburst effect.

C. Tire-track effect.

D. Radiolucent spots left ramus.

E. Right and left heavy radiolucent bands.

F. Radiopaque area.

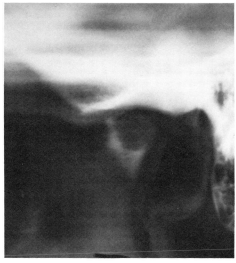

FIGURE 48   **LEFT**

CASE 48

This 55 year old female presented in the dental department of a hospital two days after sustaining a fall down a flight of stairs. Since then she has experienced some discomfort in the region of her left ear, and when she chews food she has quite marked discomfort in the left temporomandibular joint area. Examination reveals moderate tenderness to palpation over the left TMJ and slight deviation of the mandible to the left on opening movement. Occlusion is within normal limits. Routine x-ray examination of the facial skeleton revealed no apparent abnormality. Do you feel that any special x-ray examination is required?

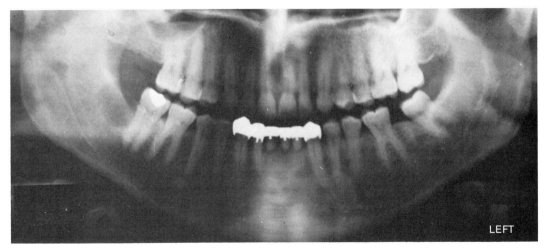

FIGURE 49A. Courtesy of Dr. Carson Mader, Washington, D.C.

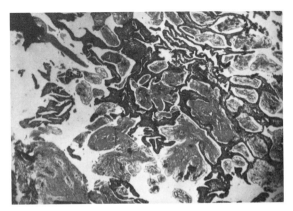

FIGURE 49B

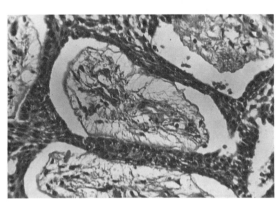

FIGURE 49C

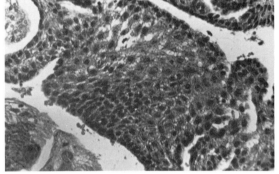

FIGURE 49D

CASE 49

The patient is a 41 year old black male. Look at the radiograph and the photomicrographs and see if you can make the diagnosis.

64

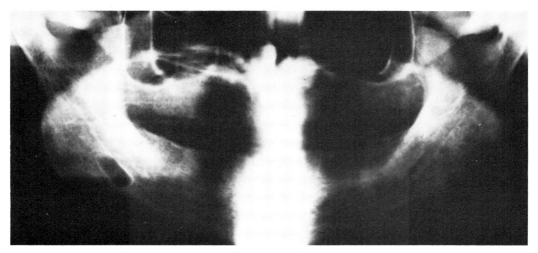

FIGURE 50A. Courtesy of Dr. Stephen Bricker, San Antonio, Texas.

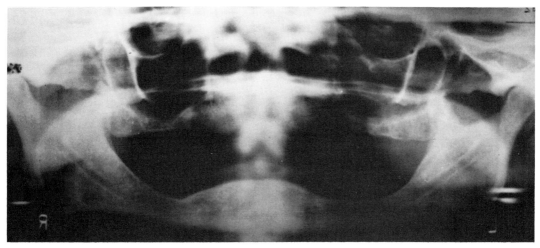

FIGURE 50B. Courtesy of Dr. James Cottone, San Antonio, Texas.

CASE 50

Both of these edentulous patients are asymptomatic, and both have the same condition, which can be diagnosed from the radiograhs alone. What is the condition?

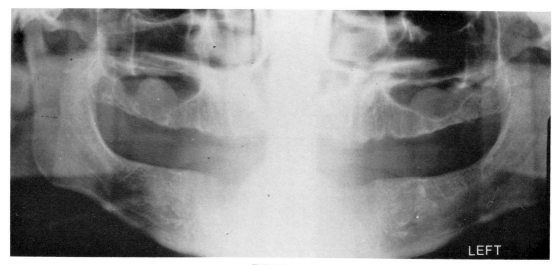

FIGURE 51

CASE 51

This patient is asymptomatic. See if you can find the affected area(s) and name the condition.

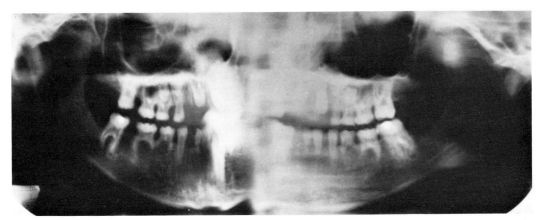

FIGURE 52

CASE 52

This eight year old patient had this radiograph taken in order to determine the extent of his condition.

QUESTIONS

1. In broad terms, what condition is depicted here?

2. What, if any, specific conditions may be characterized by this problem?

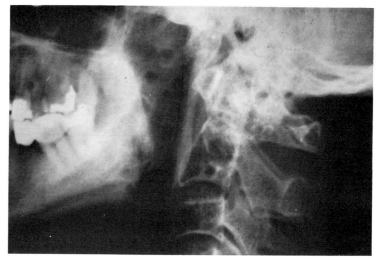

FIGURE 53A
Courtesy of Dr. Ross Hill, Montreal, Canada.

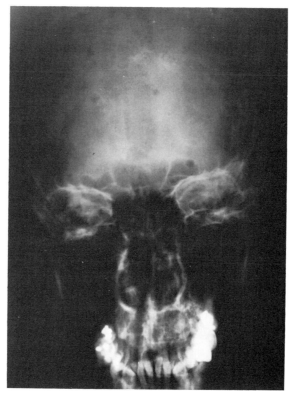

FIGURE 53B
Courtesy of Dr. Ross Hill, Montreal, Canada.

CASE 53

This 50 year old man presented in the dental clinic complaining of persistent pain in the left side of his lower jaw and a left-sided headache. He thought that this was due to a decayed molar in the left mandible. The dentist who examined the patient observed the carious molar but did not feel that this was the source of his pain. He noticed that the patient was somewhat pale, and the history had revealed malaise over the preceding few months together with a weight loss of 15 pounds. Skull films were ultimately taken and revealed this picture.

QUESTIONS

1. What do you see?

2. What is your diagnostic impression?

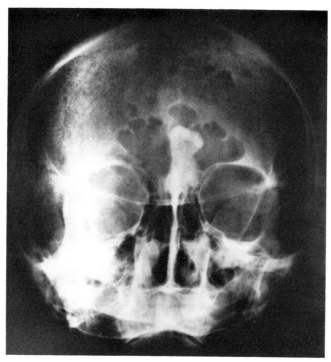

FIGURE 54
Courtesy of Dr. Ross Hill, Montreal, Canada.

CASE 54

This 62 year old edentulous female underwent a series of sinus radiographs to rule out sinusitis. This view of the frontal sinuses revealed an interesting finding.

QUESTIONS

1. What do you see?
2. What do you think this lesion is?

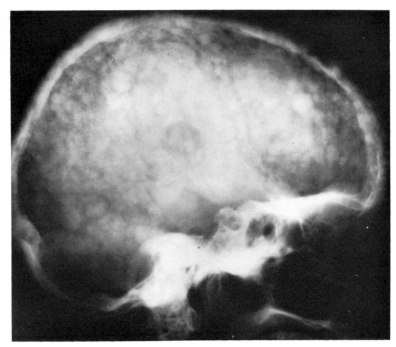

FIGURE 55

Courtesy of Dr. Ross Hill, Montreal, Canada.

CASE 55

This 45 year old man had observed the need for an increased hat size over the past few years together with some decrease in his height and bowing of his legs. Examination of the oral cavity revealed enlargement of the alveolar ridges and evidence of hypercementosis of the roots of his molar teeth. A lateral skull film revealed the picture in Figure 55. What disease do you think this patient has?

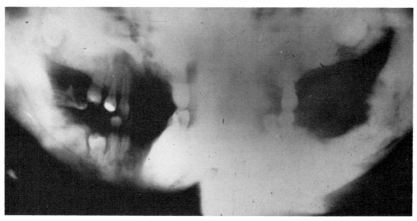

FIGURE 56A

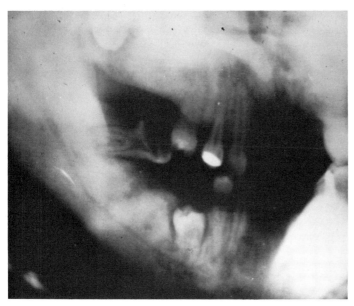

FIGURE 56B

CASE 56

This 26 year old black female has had this condition since early childhood. Most of her bones are affected, as are her jaws. She has frontal bossing and hepatosplenomegaly. There are many unerupted permanent teeth.

She is constantly being seen for chronic osteomyelitis in her jaws and has had at least one pathologic mandibular fracture. She has a low red blood (cell) count (RBC) but the serum calcium and phosphorus levels are normal as are the serum acid phosphatase and serum alkaline phosphatase levels. No other member of the family is affected.

What is your impression?

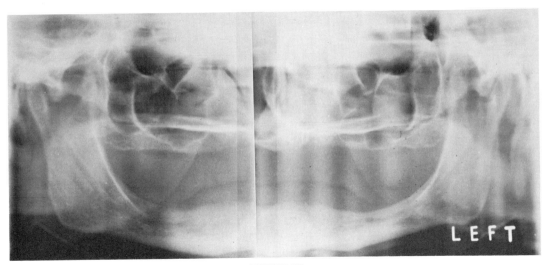

FIGURE 57

CASE 57

This 45 year old female complained of a sore throat that had been present for the past three months. She was not unduly concerned, as she had had several nagging colds and thought that this might be the tail end of them. However, for the last month she had been better, and yet the sore throat persisted. She stated that her throat was especially sore on deglutition, and she could pinpoint an area of pain on the left side of her neck just anterior to the sternomastoid muscle and below the hyoid bone.

She was not taking medication and was in good health. She had had several operations including a partial hysterectomy seven years before for a malignancy discovered from her yearly Papanicolaou (Pap) smear; she had also had her tonsils removed at the age of 12 years.

On examination, there were no tender nodes, and neither carotid body was sore on palpation.

What is your impression?

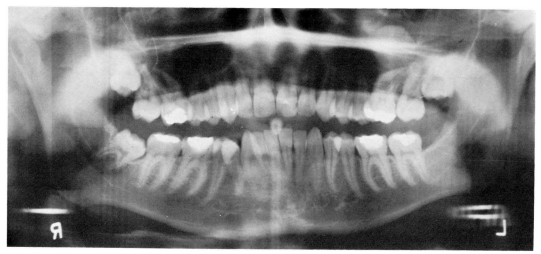

FIGURE 58. Courtesy of Dr. Tom Oliver, Montreal, Canada.

CASE 58

This 21 year old Caucasian male is asymptomatic, and this film was taken as a routine part of a new patient examination.

QUESTION

1. Once you have located the lesion, give a differential diagnosis.

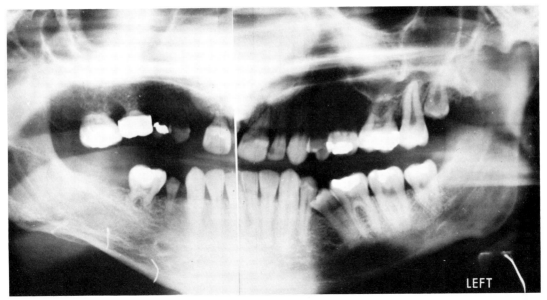

FIGURE 59A. Courtesy of Dr. Ivan Stangel and Dr. Bruce Oliver, Montreal, Canada.

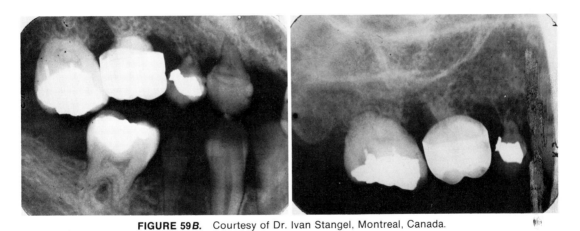

FIGURE 59B. Courtesy of Dr. Ivan Stangel, Montreal, Canada.

FIGURE 59C. Courtesy of Dr. Ivan Stangel and Dr. Bruce Oliver, Montreal, Canada.

CASE 59

This 21 year old Caucasian male received radiation therapy of the right maxillary sinus at the age of 20 months.

Two years ago, a portion of rib was grafted to the right side of his mandible. He is presently in excellent health.

QUESTION

1. What abnormalities can you detect, and what is the cause?

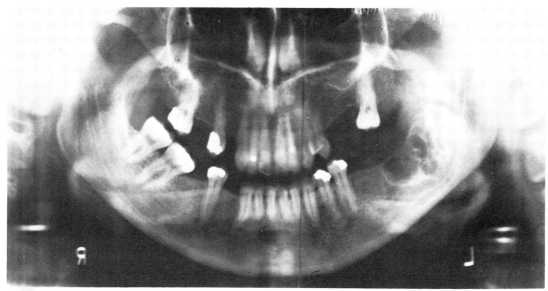

FIGURE 60A. Courtesy of Dr. Barry Sternthal, Montreal, Canada.

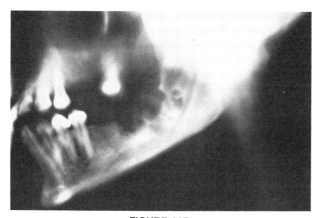

FIGURE 60B.
Courtesy of Dr. Barry Sternthal, Montreal, Canada.

CASE 60

This 38 year old Caucasian male presents with a complaint of slight pain in the left mandibular retromolar pad area and an inability to wear his partial lower denture. He has had no previous surgery other than the extraction of erupted teeth. No extractions have been performed in the last five years.

On examination, there is a firm soft-tissue swelling at the crest of the ridge in the molar area, extending down into the buccal vestibule. The tissue appears reddish and is ulcerated in one area. Figure 60B is a tomogram of the affected area.

QUESTIONS

  1. Give a differential diagnosis.

  2. What is your best choice?

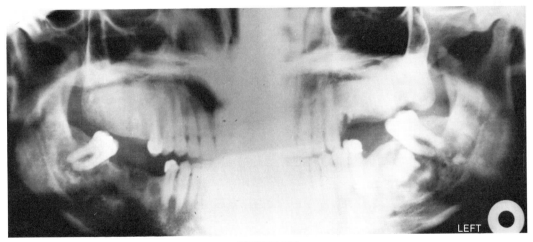

FIGURE 61A

CASE 61

This 34 year old Caucasian patient is asymptomatic. She has a firm swelling of the posterior regions on both sides of the maxilla and on the left side of the mandible.

The following data were obtained:

Calcium	10.5 mg/100 ml	(Normal 9–11.5 mg/100 ml)
Phosphorus	3.2 mg/100 ml	(Normal 3.0–4.5 mg/100 ml)
Alkaline phosphatase	14 King-Armstrong units	(Normal 5–10 King-Armstrong units)
Urinary excretion of calcium and phosphorus	Normal	
BUN	14 mg/100 ml	Normal 9–19 mg/100 ml)

The intra-oral films showed a loss of the lamina dura in most areas.

QUESTIONS

1. What is your differential diagnosis?

2. What is your definitive diagnosis?

Note. The radiolucent areas below the mandibular canal and at the inferior border on both sides are artifacts.

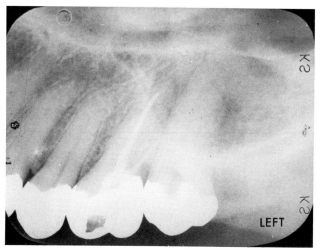

FIGURE 62A

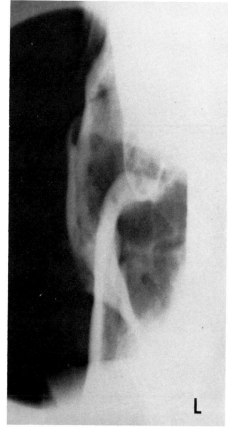

FIGURE 62B

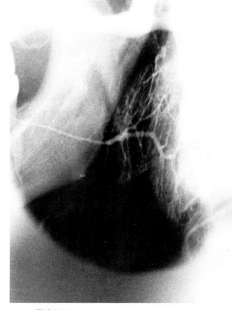

FIGURE 62C. Terminal opacification.

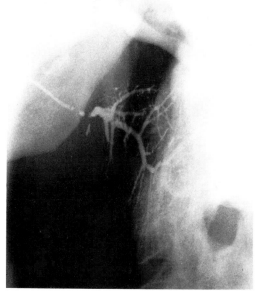

FIGURE 62D. 15-minute emptying.

CASE 62

Mrs. Debit, a long-time patient of Dr. Freeze, presented to the office with pain in the left temporomandibular joint area and swelling in the left cheek. The pain had begun six months earlier while she was vacationing in California, and endodontic treatment was completed on the upper left first permanent molar (Fig. 62*A*). After her vacation, the symptoms and periodic swelling persisted. At times she was febrile. Her physician-employer gave her penicillin, which would reduce the fever for a short time, but it always recurred. During the previous six weeks, the pain in the left TMJ region had become more pronounced. At times, the pain radiated to the ear and down the neck, and all of the teeth on the left side were tender. Propoxyphene relieved the pain, but a heating pad applied to the cheek did not reduce the swelling. Past medical history elicited a fracture of the left condyle 12 years earlier. The extra-oral examination revealed that the patient had a mild, nontender swelling of the left cheek. There was no other swelling, mass, or tenderness to palpation. The intra-oral examination revealed normal hard and soft tissues, while the salivary flow from the left parotid duct was clear but reduced in quantity. There was no stenosis or evidence of trauma at the left parotid papilla. A transorbital radiograph of the left condyle revealed a united but medially rotated left condylar head due to the previous fracture (Fig. 62*B*). A left parotid sialogram was performed, and the results may be seen in Figure 62*C* – terminal opacification phase and Figure 62*D* – 15-minute emptying film.

QUESTIONS

1. Describe the 15-minute sialograph.
2. What is your diagnosis?

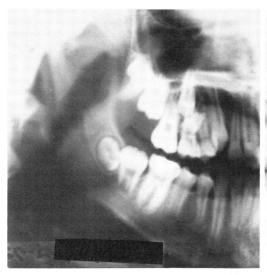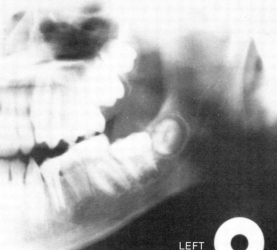

FIGURE 63

CASE 63

This 11 year old girl of Chinese origin presented to her dentist for a routine check-up. He noted delayed eruption of the maxillary right second bicuspid; the other three second bicuspids were present. Additionally, the upper right second deciduous molar was not mobile, and a small, firm nodule was palpable in the buccal vestibule above this tooth.

This film was taken in order to determine the cause of the delayed eruption.

QUESTION

1. What is your impression? Try to give a differential diagnosis.

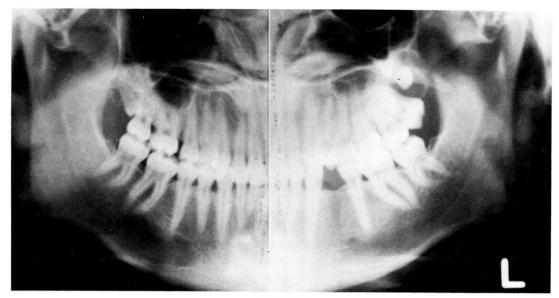

FIGURE 64

CASE 64

This 23 year old Caucasian female is asymptomatic. What is your interpretation of this routine film?

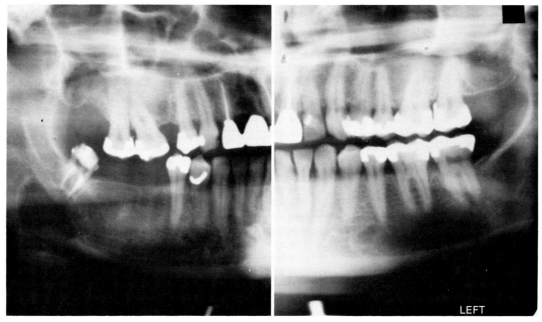

FIGURE 65

CASE 65

This 32 year old male Caucasian patient fell off his motorcycle and subsequently developed a "sore jaw." Part of the radiographic examination included the panoramic film seen here. The pain was confined to the right cheek. There were no other signs or symptoms, except that the pain was worse when he masticated food.

As the consultant on this case, what notable radiographic findings would you report? Include all areas of interest.

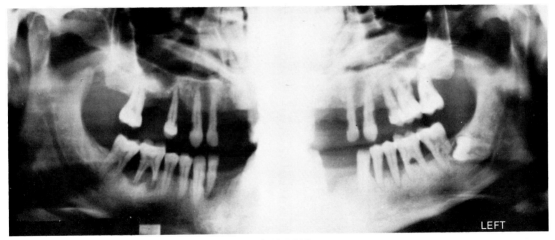

FIGURE 66A

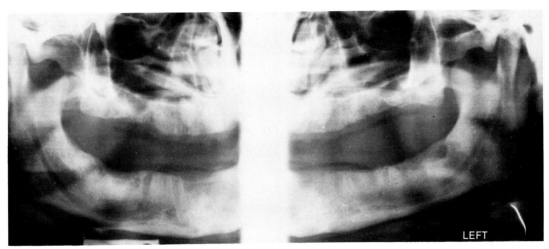

FIGURE 66B

CASE 66

This 49 year old male of East Indian origin first presented with severe periodontal disease (Fig. 66A).

All of his teeth were extracted, and complete upper and lower dentures were constructed. At the six-month follow-up, the radiograph seen in Figure 66B was taken.

QUESTIONS

1. What is your impression of the radiolucency seen in the left mandibular third molar region?

2. Give a differential diagnosis and your recommendations for obtaining a definitive diagnosis.

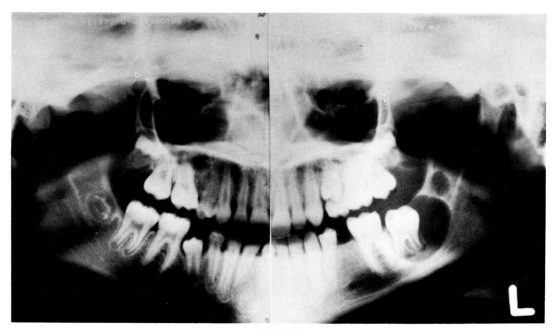

FIGURE 67

CASE 67

This 12 year old girl was raised in a community with a fluoridated water supply and had never required dental treatment. She had received routine check-ups and fluoride treatments since the age of three years.

The patient suddenly developed pain in the left mandibular molar area. There was some trismus. On examination, the mucosa on the crest of the ridge distal to the first molar was red, swollen, and ulcerated. The upper second molar was traumatizing this area.

Looking at this radiograph, what findings would you report in the left mandible?

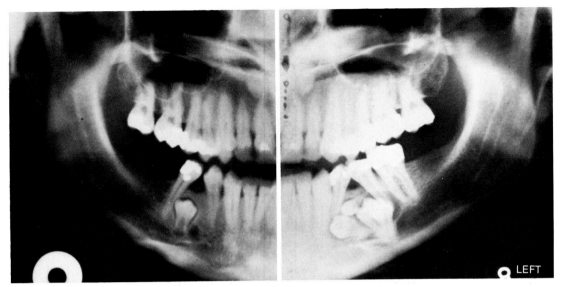

FIGURE 68

CASE 68

This is a 22 year old Caucasian male who is asymptomatic.

QUESTIONS

    1. Based on the radiograph alone, what would you report?

    2. What is your impression?

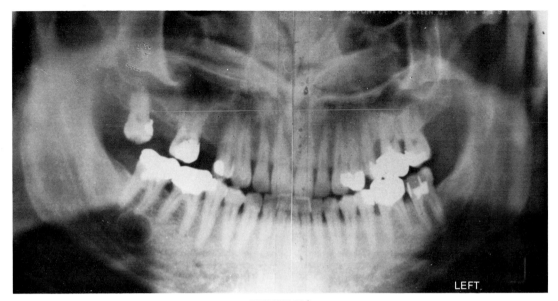

FIGURE 69A

CASE 69

This is an asymptomatic patient with a nonvital lower right second molar.

QUESTIONS

1. Give a description of the lesion in question.
2. Give a differential diagnosis.

A duplicate radiograph is included in the answer section.

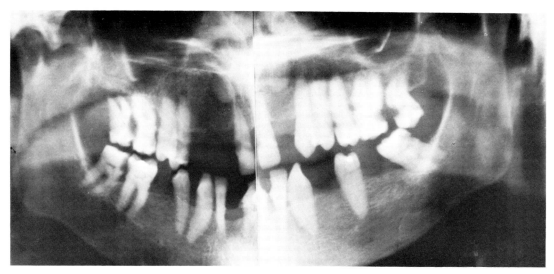

FIGURE 70   LEFT

CASE 70

This patient has a history of sore throat of six weeks' duration. He was given an antibiotic initially, with temporary relief. Examination subsequently revealed a large indurated mass occupying the right tonsillar fossa, involving the anterior pillar, as well as a large, palpable, mobile, nontender node in the midcervical region on the same side. Oral hygiene is poor; there is moderate to severe periodontal disease; and there are a number of moderately large carious lesions present.

QUESTIONS

1. What dental treatment would you suggest? (Keep in mind the probable mode of therapy for the mass.)

2. What other radiographic findings would you report?

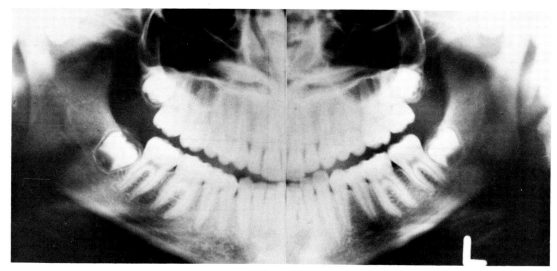

FIGURE 71A

CASE 71

This 15 year old Caucasian girl had no complaints when she was seen for her routine check-up. As a matter of routine for new patients, this panoramic film was taken.

There was no history of trauma, and all the teeth responded positively to the electric pulp test.

QUESTIONS

1. Where is the lesion?

2. Give a differential diagnosis.

3. Would you make your final recommendations to the patient, based on the information given?

4. Name the artifact seen in the periapical view in the answer section.

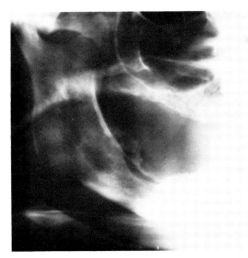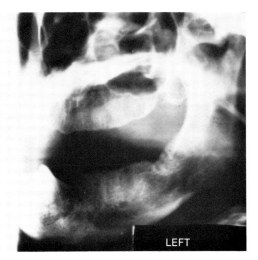

FIGURE 72A

CASE 72

This 56 year old Caucasian male patient had radiation therapy nine years ago for a carcinoma of the posterior third of the right lateral border of the tongue. The patient is a chronic alcoholic and has a previous history of pulmonary tuberculosis. He smokes two packs of cigarettes per day.

When Figure 72A was taken, the patient's complaint was one of increasing pain over the previous two months, ever since a root tip had been removed from the right mandibular molar area. The patient was wearing full upper and lower dentures.

QUESTIONS

1. What is your impression?

2. What is the cause of this condition?

3. How could this have been prevented?

4. How would you treat this case?

Note. A periapical radiograph of the affected area may be seen in the answer section.

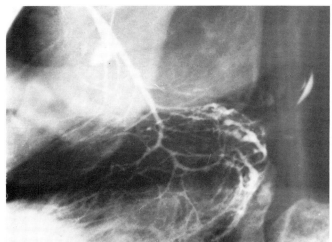

FIGURE 73A

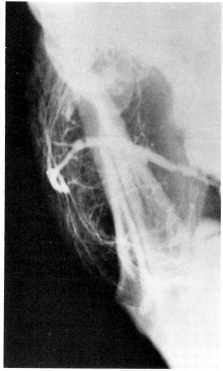

FIGURE 73B

CASE 73

This 64 year old Caucasian male patient was completely unaware of a swelling behind the right angle of the mandible, which was found at the time of a routine dental check-up.

On further examination, a mass was palpated along the posterior border of the right ramus of the mandible. This was firm, indurated, and slightly fixed. The lesion was nontender and appeared to be causing slight elevation of the right ear lobe. No palpable lymph nodes were detected, and intra-orally, some fullness in the right lateral wall of the pharynx was detected.

After viewing the sialogram, what is your impression?

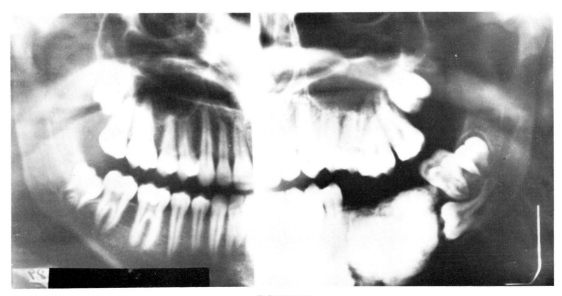

FIGURE 74

CASE 74

This 15 year old boy presented with a five-year history of intermittent, moderate pain in the left body of the mandible. The patient had become aware of a deformity of the lateral and inferior aspects of the midbody of the mandible. There was no paresthesia of the lower lip on the left side.

Clinical examination revealed a mass expanding the buccal and inferior aspects of the left body of the mandible, and the mucosa overlying the edentulous area was tender to palpation.

The lesion was excised locally. The presence of an enamel matrix was identified on histologic examination.

QUESTIONS

1. What is the most likely diagnosis?

2. What other, more aggressive lesion with these characteristics should the clinician be on the lookout for?

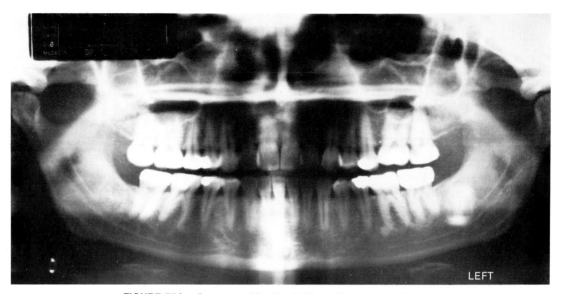

FIGURE 75A. Courtesy of Dr. David Blair, St. Lambert, Canada.

CASE 75

This 24 year old black female, in excellent systemic health, gave a history of having had all four of her third molars removed 14 months ago. She was asymptomatic, and this panoramic film was taken as part of a routine new-patient screening procedure.

What is your impression? Now, if you wish, you may consult a second panoramic film taken two weeks later, which is shown in the answer section. Take a few moments, and ascertain that you've looked everywhere.

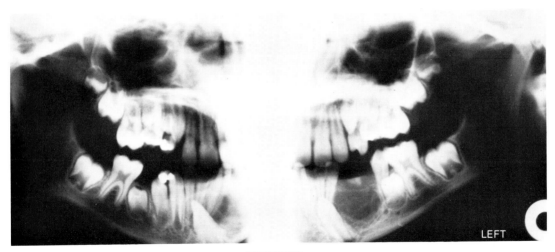

FIGURE 76

CASE 76

Janet Toothfairy, a 10 year old Caucasian female, reported to her family dentist one day for a routine check-up. The bite-wing films revealed a possible missing left mandibular first bicuspid, and the bone in this area had an unusual appearance. There was no history of trauma and no symptomatology. At this time, the panoramic film seen in Figure 76 was taken.

QUESTIONS

1. Describe the radiographic appearance of the lesion.

2. Give a differential diagnosis.

3. Considering age, sex, location, and radiographic evidence, what is your most likely choice?

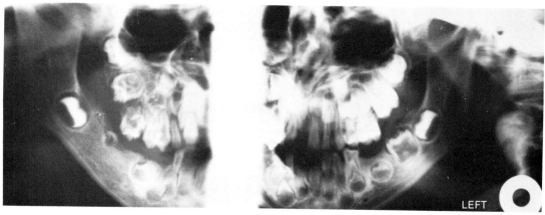

FIGURE 77A. Age 8.

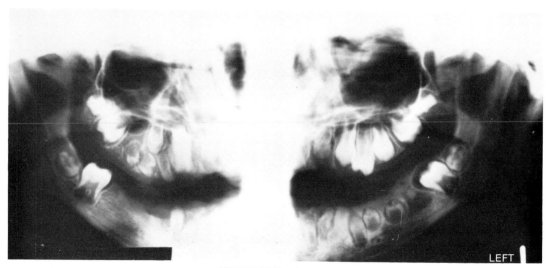

FIGURE 77B. Age 12.

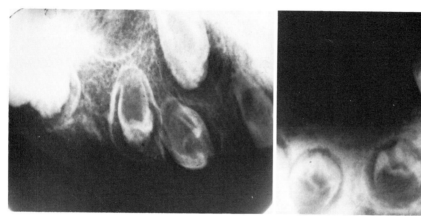

FIGURE 77C. Age 12.   **FIGURE 77D.** Age 8.

CASE 77

This six year old patient of Greek origin reported to the emergency clinic with swelling and pain in the right body of the mandible (Fig. 77A). It was found that the ridge was being traumatized by the upper second deciduous molar, which appeared severely hypoplastic clinically and had many sharp, jagged edges. Several extractions were performed at this time and all the deciduous teeth had been extracted by the time the patient was 11 years old. As none of the permanent teeth had erupted, complete upper and lower dentures were constructed. Figure 77B shows the patient, at age 12 years, with no permanent teeth erupted.

This patient had multiple congenital malformations. At age two years, they consisted of capillary hemangiectasis of the face and neck, hypertelorism, corneal opacities, bilateral dermolipomas of the lateral bulbar conjunctiva of both eyes, and bilateral chorioretinal atrophy. The skull films revealed sclerosis in both frontal bones and sclerotic changes in the petrous pyramids as well as dense calcifications in the left side of the neck. The remainder of the skeletal survey was normal.

QUESTIONS

1. What congenital defect appears to be affecting the deciduous teeth (Fig. 77A)?

2. What congenital defect appears to be affecting some permanent teeth (Figs. 77B, 77C, and 77D)?

3. Can you name the syndrome?

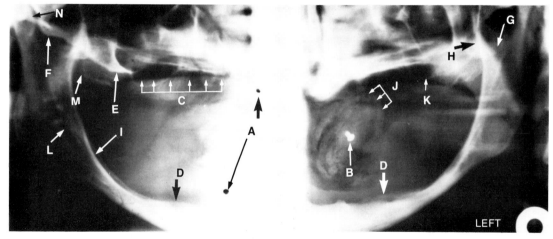

FIGURE 78

CASE 78

This 64 year old patient presented with pain and some swelling in the right body of the mandible and a sensation of pins and needles in the right lower lip. He denied a history of trauma but stated that the pain and swelling had been present for five days.

QUESTIONS

1. What is your diagnosis?

2. Give a differential diagnosis for the radiopaque objects seen at the right ramus of the mandible.

3. Identify arrows A through N.

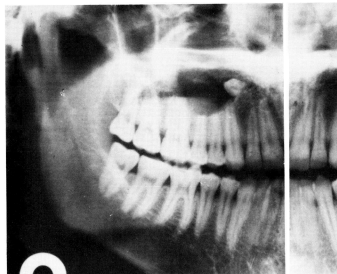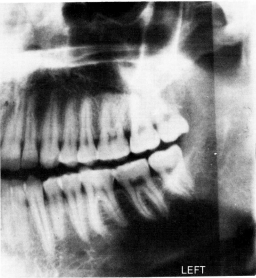

FIGURE 79A

CASE 79

1. Give a differential diagnosis for the radiopacity in the right maxillary sinus of this 28 year old patient.

2. What is your first choice? Describe the radiographic findings that suggest this. (You may wish to consult the periapical film in the answer section.)

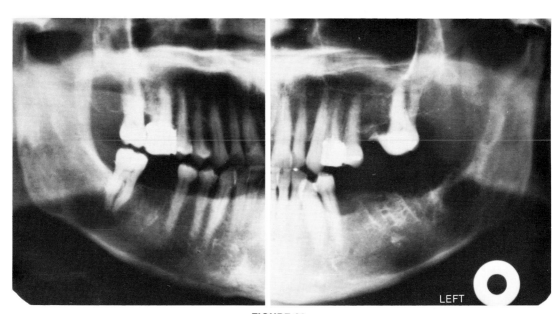

FIGURE 80

CASE 80

This 52 year old Caucasian male patient was first seen for pain in the left mandible. The patient revealed that he had had two molars extracted six weeks before, and after many visits to his dentist for persistent pain, he was referred to the hospital facial pain clinic for further evaluation.

At the time of examination, the extraction sites of the lower left molar teeth were tender when explored and contained some purulent material. There appeared to be some buccal expansion of the posterior aspect of the mandible, and there was slight trismus. Oral hygiene was poor; the patient was emaciated, smoked two packs of cigarettes per day and had recently joined Alcoholics Anonymous. There was slight paresthesia of the lower left lip. Except for edematous, reddish gingiva at the extraction site, the soft tissue in the area appeared normal.

The patient had not had a medical examination in many years and had never had any major surgery. He complained of a persistent, nonproductive cough. He further revealed an increasing dyspnea over the past six months.

What is your impression as to the cause of the jaw pain?

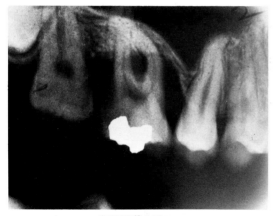

FIGURE 81A1

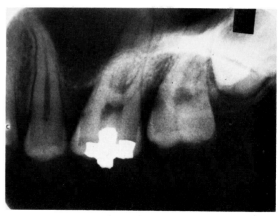

FIGURE 81A2

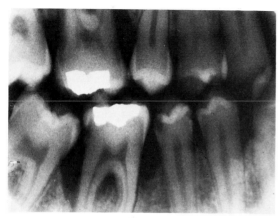

FIGURE 81A3

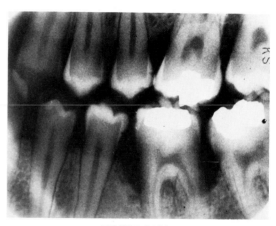

FIGURE 81A4

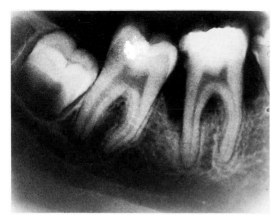

FIGURE 81A5

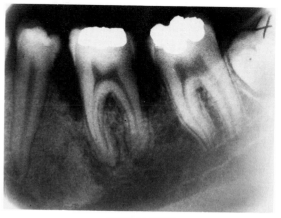

FIGURE 81A6

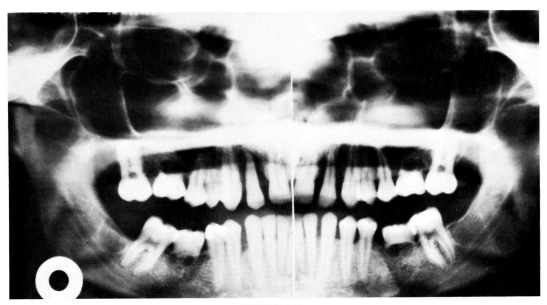

FIGURE 81B

CASE 81

This 17 year old female, originally from Barbados, was referred for diagnosis and treatment of a rather alarming loss of bone around the first molars. This condition was discovered in the routine bite-wing examination (Figs. 81A3 and 81A4).

On examination, it was found that oral hygiene was poor, moderate caries was present, but clinically, the gingiva appeared surprisingly healthy in all areas. Deep pockets were found about all four first molars, and there were 4-mm pockets around both maxillary lateral incisors (Fig. 81B).

The systemic work-up showed the patient to be in excellent general health.

The treatment consisted of amalgam restorations, scaling and curettage of the pockets around the maxillary lateral incisors, extraction of all the first molars, and transplantation of developing third molars into the extraction sites. Figure 81B shows the transplanted teeth in place 10 months postoperatively, just after removal of the ligature wires. Figure 81C is a four-year follow-up.

QUESTIONS

1. What is your diagnosis?

2. Comment on the success or failure of the treatment.

3. What changes have occurred in the transplanted teeth over the past four years?

Illustration continued on following page.

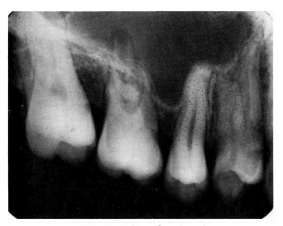

FIGURE 81C1 *(Continued)*

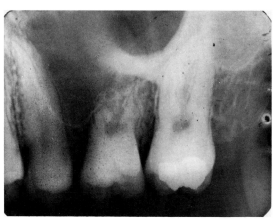

FIGURE 81C2 *(Continued)*

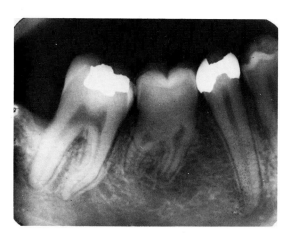

FIGURE 81C3 *(Continued)*

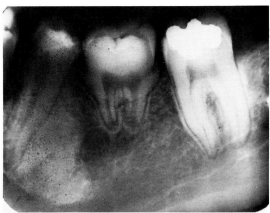

FIGURE 81C4 *(Continued)*

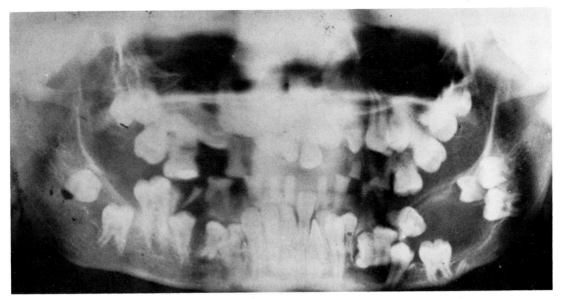

FIGURE 82A

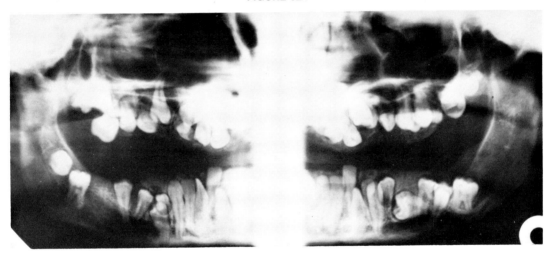

FIGURE 82B

CASE 82

This 16 year old male Caucasian adolescent presented to the clinic with a complaint of toothache. His mother expressed concern over the prolonged retention of his deciduous teeth and stated that this was causing her son to have progressively worsening psychologic problems.

A complete skeletal survey was performed. Many skull abnormalities were reported, including wormian bones and open fontanelles. The clavicles were markedly underdeveloped bilaterally, and there was clinodactyly in the fourth digits bilaterally. Slight scoliosis was present.

Figure 82A shows the patient as he first presented, while Figure 82B shows the patient nine months after all deciduous teeth and some impacted permanent teeth were extracted. The large radiolucent area in the left mandible was also managed surgically and proved to be a follicular cyst.

To help with the psychologic problems, which were by now severe, complete upper and lower dentures were constructed. The patient was subsequently lost to follow-up.

What was his condition?

103

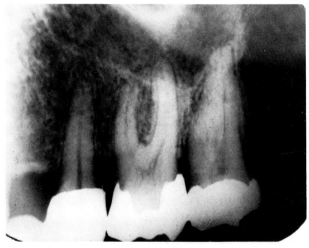

FIGURE 83A1

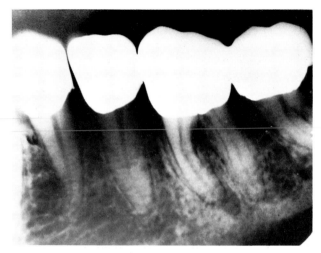

FIGURE 83A2

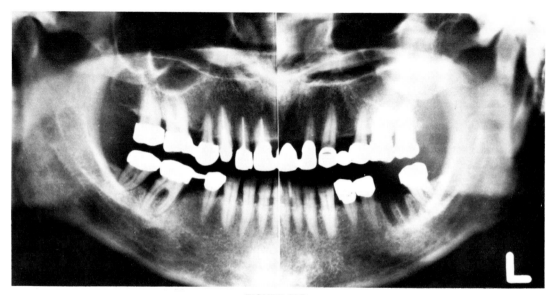

FIGURE 83B

CASE 83

This 55 year old female of Polish origin presented with burning pain in the left mandibular posterior area. She complained of chronic pain on and off over the past six months. She reported that she had recently lost 15 pounds and attributed this to her inability to eat properly when she was in pain. Her vital signs were normal. The physical examination revealed nothing contributory, and the chest film was normal. She had no history of previous major surgery.

The radiographs in Figures 83*A1* and 83*A2* were taken, and the lower left first molar was extracted. The patient continued to have persistent pain over the next three weeks and complained that it now seemed generalized over the entire left side of the face. At this time, a panoramic radiograph was taken (Fig. 83*B*).

QUESTIONS

1. Do you think the pain was arising from the extraction socket?

2. What important radiographic finding has been overlooked? Explain.

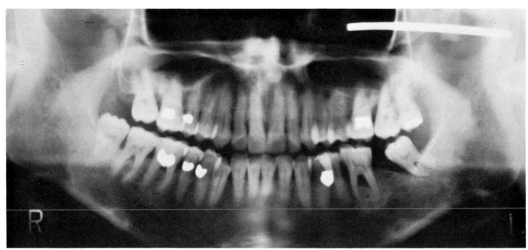

FIGURE 84. Courtesy of Dr. Charles Morris and Mr. Felix Cardero, San Antonio, Texas.   **LEFT**

CASE 84

1. With the use of this radiograph, compare and contrast the development of the periodontal condition affecting the mandibular left first molar and the periodontal condition affecting the mandibular left third molar.

2. How could these conditions have been prevented?

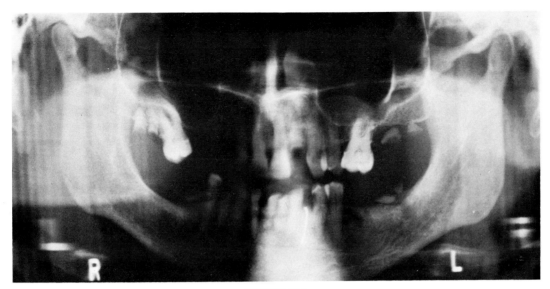

FIGURE 85A

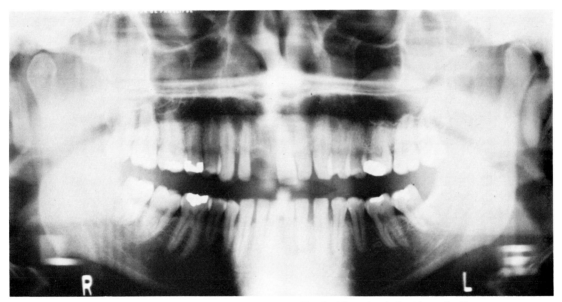

FIGURE 85B. Figure 85, *A* and *B* courtesy of Dr. Olaf Langland, San Antonio, Texas.

CASE 85

1. Describe the status of the soft tissue lining the floor of the left maxillary sinus in each radiograph.

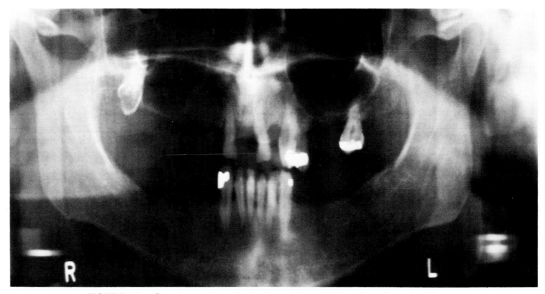

FIGURE 86. Courtesy of Leo Bedock and Don Adkins, San Antonio, Texas.

CASE 86

1. Identify the condition present in the right maxilla of this 47 year old, otherwise healthy, Caucasian female.

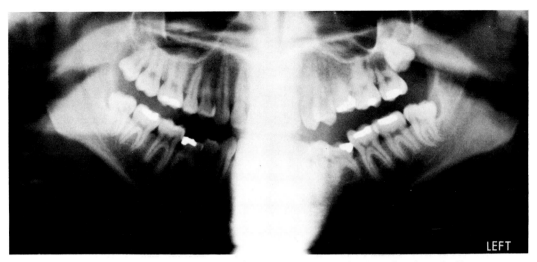

FIGURE 87. Courtesy of Dr. Charles Morris and Mr. Felix Cardero, San Antonio, Texas.

CASE 87

This 22 year old Caucasian female presented with a complaint of pain in the mandibular left posterior area. There was trismus and a low-grade fever. Tender, freely mobile nodes were palpable in both the right and left submaxillary areas.

QUESTIONS

    1. What is your diagnosis?

    2. What congenital defect is present?
Substantiate your answers radiographically!

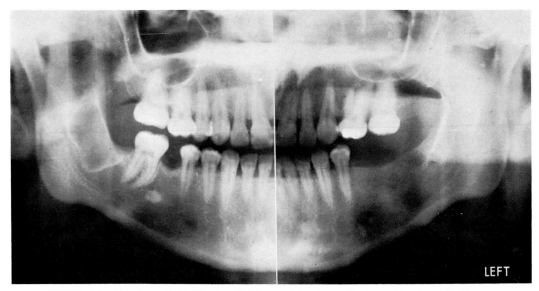

FIGURE 88. Courtesy of Dr. Stephen Bricker and Dr. James Cottone, San Antonio, Texas.

CASE 88

This 25 year old Caucasian female had her impacted mandibular right third molar extracted six years ago. A well-developed follicular cyst was excised at that time, but neither the tooth nor the tissue was submitted for pathologic examination. The current lesion was excised. At the time of operation, some white, curdy material was noted and the histopathologic report described epithelium that was arranged in a "corrugated" pattern.

QUESTIONS

1. What is your impression?

ANSWERS

CASE 1

Periapical cemental dysplasia (multiple cementomas).

CASE 2

1. Differential diagnosis:
    a). *Cyclic neutropenia.*
    b). *Agranulocytosis.*
    c). *Juvenile diabetes.*
    d). *Papillon-Lefèvre syndrome.*
    e). *Hypophosphatasia.*
    f). *Juvenile periodontosis.*
    g). *Scurvy.*
2. *Cyclic neutropenia* would be a good possibility. The patient has a history of chronic infections. The clue here is that neutrophil counts were obtained at timed intervals, and at no time was the white blood (cell) count (WBC) depressed beyond normal limits. *Agranulocytosis* would also be a good possibility, but note that the WBCs were within normal limits. Note also that agranulocytosis is often, though not always, associated with the chronic intake of drugs that have a depressant effect on bone marrow production of white blood cells. The patient was not taking any drugs at the time of examination. *Juvenile diabetes* is often associated with chronic infection and periodontal disease in children. Note, however, that the glucose tolerance test and the fasting blood sugar (glucose) (FBS) were normal. *Papillon-Lefèvre syndrome* is associated with early onset of periodontal disease. Note, however, that palmar-plantar hyperkeratosis was not reported, and there was no calcification in the falx cerebri. *Hypophosphatasia* is associated with the early shedding of deciduous teeth, but note that alkaline phosphatase levels were normal. *Juvenile periodontosis*, though it cannot be diagnosed definitely, is the best choice, especially in the absence of all systemic disorders.

Comment. Note that the elevated erythrocyte sedimentation rate (ESR) is a nonspecific finding and is often elevated in children, especially when infection is present. Although scurvy is a relatively rare condition, note that there should be abundant natural vitamin C from the citrus fruits that the mother included in the child's diet. Another interesting point is the resistance of the oral flora to penicillin, erythromycin, and tetracycline. The frequency with which this child was given antibiotics for upper respiratory tract infections, tonsillitits, and earaches has probably contributed to the development of these resistant strains of oral flora.

This child was eventually hospitalized with pneumonia. During this time, he received regular monitoring with daily hemograms. Within a 10-day period, his WBCs plummeted to 2600, to 3400, and to 4600, with normal WBCs in between.

FINAL DIAGNOSIS: Cyclic Neutropenia.

CASE 3

1. Differential diagnosis:

This is an interesting case because there are two sets of differential diagnoses. The first is based on the radiographs and consists of :

a). *Fibrous dysplasia.*
b). *Paget's disease of bone.*
c). *Hyperparathyroidism (primary or secondary).*

The second is based on the detailed histopathologic examination of the biopsy specimen and consists of:

a). *Fibrous dysplasia.*
b). *Giant cell granuloma.*
c). *Osteomalacia.*
d). *Paget's disease of bone.*

2. The definitive diagnosis consists of correlating radiographic and histopathologic findings with the laboratory investigation and previous medial history. Note that the patient's serum calcium level is high normal but the serum phosphorus level is decreased and the serum alkaline phosphatase level is increased. The urinary excretion of calcium is also increased. The urinary excretion of hydroxyproline is simply an indication of an increased degradation of collagenous bone matrix. These findings are consistent with a diagnosis of *secondary hyperparathyroidism.* Note that the secondary hyperparathyroidism develops as a result of increased urinary excretion of calcium, producing decreased serum calcium levels. This results in increased production of parathyroid hormone (PTH), bone resorption, and re-establishment of high normal serum calcium levels. Note that the increased urinary excretion of calcium is a sequela of the chronic renal disease, and unlike the elevated serum calcium levels seen in primary hyperparathyroidism, the serum calcium levels seen in secondary hyperparathyroidism are often normal to high normal.

3. There is a marked *narrowing and/or obliteration of the pulp chambers and root canals* inconsistent with the young age of the patient. In Figures 3A, 3B, 3C, there is a *generalized loss of the lamina dura* and a *"ground-glass" appearance of the alveolar bone.* In Figures 3D and 3E, *a radiolucent lesion* has developed about the apex of the lower left first molar. There is an associated *resorption of the root tips* and *extrusion* of the mandibular left first molar.

1. Differential diagnosis:
   a). *Ameloblastoma.*
   b). *Pindborg tumor.*
   c). *Aneurysmal bone cyst.*
   d). *Central giant cell granuloma.*
   e). *Odontogenic myxoma.*

2. The age of the patient, the location, and the soap bubble appearance of the lesion are typical of the *ameloblastoma*. The clue, however, is the fairly radical procedure that was carried out. Remember that the ameloblastoma has a relatively high recurrence rate, and when the lesion is as extensive as this, conservative therapy is contraindicated. The other lesions could have been treated conservatively.

CASE 5

1. *Every's syndrome.* Pain caused by buccally erupting third molars.

2. *Cleidocranial dysplasia. Gardner's syndrome.*

CASE 6

1. Differential diagnosis:

LESION	SALIENT FEATURES
a). *Primordial cyst.*	Note that the first primary molar is present with no replacement.
b). *Aneurysmal bone cyst.*	Note the multilocular, honeycomb appearance of the lesion. This often occurs in young patients.
c). *Central giant cell granuloma.*	Note the multilocular, honeycomb appearance of the lesion. This often occurs in children and adolescents.
d). *Ameloblastic fibroma.*	The location, age, and radiographic appearance are typical.
e). *Garré's osteomyelitis.*	The age and expansile nature of the lesion are typical. A history of pulpal involvement of the first primary molar or trauma would be helpful.
f). *Traumatic cyst.*	The expansion as observed on the occlusal view is often seen. The lesion is usually unilocular and may, though not commonly, be associated with divergence of roots. The age of the patient is typical for this lesion.

2. *Central ossifying (or cementifying) fibroma.* For the more typical appearance of this lesion, refer to Figure 37.

CASE 7

Primary hyperparathyroidism. First, note the biopsy specimen. The lesion is typical of a central giant cell granuloma. Note that the serum phosphorus level is decreased, while the serum calcium level is just slightly elevated. Repeated tests eventually revealed a serum calcium level of 11.9 mg/100 ml. These data suggest a diagnosis of *primary hyperparathyroidism.* In secondary hyperparathyroidism, there is usually a history of renal disease and increased urinary excretion of calcium on a low-calcium diet, while the serum calcium level remains high normal. The hypochromic, microcytic anemia is secondary to chronic blood loss from the mass.

The patient was explored for a parathyroid tumor, and a parathyroid adenoma was removed. The patient developed hypocalcemia (calcium level was 7 mg/100 ml) postoperatively, and calcium gluconate was administered intravenously. The tingling in her fingers and the positive Chvostek's sign subsided, and she was discharged on medications of vitamins C and D, calcium lactate, and ferrous sulfate.

CASE 8

1. Differential diagnosis:
    a). *Peripheral giant cell granuloma.*
    b). *Pyogenic granuloma.*
    c). *Peripheral odontogenic fibroma.*
    d). *Squamous cell carcinoma.*
    e). *Other malignancy.*

2. The gingival biopsy specimen revealed that the subepithelial connective tissue was occupied by sheets of round, large, basophilic cells, resembling reticulum cells. There were numerous larger, multinucleated cells with pale cytoplasms. There were also numerous mitotic figures, and a few plasma cells were present. These findings are compatible with a diagnosis of *reticulum cell sarcoma.*

CASE 9

1. Differential diagnosis:
    a). *Periapical or residual cyst.*
    b). *Primordial cyst.*
    c). *Metastatic prostatic carcinoma.*
    d). *Ameloblastoma.*
    e). *Mucoepidermoid carcinoma.*

FINAL DIAGNOSIS: This case proved to be *mucoepidermoid carcinoma.* Note that this is the common location for a central mucoepidermoid carcinoma and that sometimes a clear mucous fluid can be aspirated.

CASE 10

1. *Osteoradionecrosis.*
2. The following factors are required in order to develop this condition:
   a). *Radiation (therapeutic levels)*
   b). *Trauma.*
   c). *Inflammation.*

CASE 11

The radiograph reveals normally erupting maxillary third molars. The mandibular third molars are not seen. The mandibular first molars are missing, and both mandibular second bicuspids have migrated posteriorly and have become distally impacted against the mesial roots of both mandibular second molars.

There is evidence that suggests a history of trauma to the maxillary central incisors, and the apices of teeth numbers 11 and 21 appear normal. The remainder of the dentition appears normal. Bitewing and visual examinations are required to rule out further caries as well as to establish the periodontal status of the patient.

Comment. Note that unerupted teeth *"migrate"* distally, whereas posterior movement of erupted teeth is referred to as distal *"drift."* Both *distal drift* and *distal migration* are exceptions to the rule, the more common movement of teeth being toward the mesial.

CASE 12

1. This patient's age is 10 years — plus or minus one year.

Comment. Note that the 12-year molar has not yet erupted but that the mandibular first bicuspid appears to have erupted; therefore, the patient is at least 10 years of age.

2. The mandibular second premolar appears to be erupting *buccally.*

Comment. Note that this lateral jaw view was taken by placing the film cassette against the involved side of the face. The object closest to the film will appear the most opaque when compared with objects of similar density. Note that the tooth in question is slightly more opaque than its neighbors, therefore it is erupting buccally.

This impression can be confirmed by the use of the buccal object rule (Clark's rule) or by taking an occlusal view.

3. The radiographic findings are compatible with a *follicular cyst* associated with the erupting mandibular second premolar. In addition, the relatively large size of the cyst suggests the possibility that it is of the keratocyst type. If this is the case, the "jaw cyst–basal cell nevus-bifid rib" syndrome (Gorlin-Goltz syndrome) should be ruled out. Note also that the odontogenic keratocyst has a propensity for recurrence and usually does so within five years postoperatively.

CASE 13

1. Differential diagnosis:
   a). *Antrolith.*
   b). *Osteoma* arising from the posterior wall of the maxillary sinus.
   c). *Retained root tip.*

2. The *retained root tip* is the most likely choice because of the root-like shape of the object and the presence of what appears to be a root canal.

CASE 14

The radiolucency was in fact a *residual cyst.*

Comment. Note that the lesion appears to have perforated in the ramus area. In addition, the large size of the area, along with a slightly scalloped outline, suggests a type of keratocyst.

The epithelium in the biopsy specimen was not keratinized, nor was there a "corrugated" pattern. The patient had an unremarkable recovery after surgery.

CASE 15

1. The *maxillary left central incisor.*

2. If the tooth is nonvital, treatment should consist of *occlusal equilibration, curettage,* and *endodontic therapy.* In actual fact, there was a 10-mm pocket on the palatal side of the tooth and a 5-mm pocket on the labial aspect. The tooth was nonvital. Also, note the wear on the opposing mandibular lateral incisor in Figure 15A.

After equilibration, local curettage, and endodontic therapy, the tooth stabilized and the periapical area resolved. A 5-mm pocket remained around the tooth. The prognosis remained guarded.

3. Bilateral maxillary *peg laterals.*

4. The *mandibular left second molar* has the poorest prognosis, owing to *mesial tipping* and a mesial "pseudo pocket" that has developed into a true pocket that appears to extend almost to the apex.

CASE 16

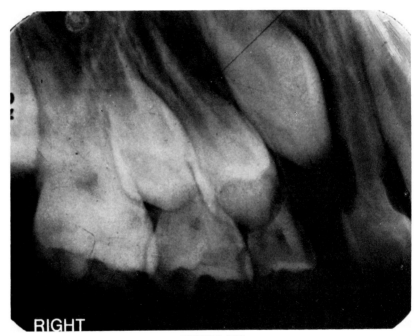

FIGURE 16B

1. The *maxillary right lateral incisor.*
2. This treatment was subsequently performed because of the *excessive resorption of the root* of tooth number 12. The area was curetted, and no significant pathosis was reported. The cause of the resorption was probably pressure caused by the impaction of the erupting canine tooth.

Comment. Note that a lesion associated with tooth resorption, especially in a young patient, is an ominous sign and should not be ignored. Considering the patient's age and the location of the lesion, several possibilities are

a). *Eosinophilic granuloma–histiocytosis X group.*
b). *Odontogenic adenomatoid tumor.*
c). *Fibrosarcoma.*

1. *Removal of the mandibular right third molar,* which is mesially impacted.

2. Differential diagnosis:
   a). *Benign cementoblastoma.*
   b). *Periapical cemental dysplasia.*
   c). *Chronic diffuse sclerosing osteomyelitis.*

Comment. The radiographic features of the *benign cemento-blastoma* are usually pathognomonic. The lesion usually grows equally in all directions; it is delineated by a radiolucent area; and usually the outline of the root is lost within the lesion. The tooth is vital, and the lesion most often involves mandibular posterior teeth. The lesion is often seen in young people and is often solitary.

In this case, the patient is 45 years old, and she is black. *Periapical cemental dysplasia* is common among this group, and the lesions may be multiple. Note that in this radiograph, there are several other radiopaque areas, including teeth numbers 17 and 37, protruding into the maxillary sinus. Note also the periapical radiolucencies at the apices of teeth numbers 32, 34, and 35 and possibly of teeth numbers 41 and 42. Except for number 35, these teeth are vital. These findings are compatible with a diagnosis of *multiple cementomas.*

Note, however, that this middle-aged black female has periodontal disease, heavy calculus, and several associated nutrient canals in the lower anterior area. These findings are often seen in *chronic diffuse sclerosing osteomyelitis.*

3. Other pathologic processes seen in the radiograph:
   a). *Caries:* occlusal — tooth number 18; distal — tooth number 17; mesial—tooth number 11; mesial—tooth number 21; mesial—tooth number 26; and distal—tooth number 35.

Note. This kind of radiograph cannot be used exclusively for the diagnosis of caries.
   b). *A periapical radiolucent area* of tooth number 35 with a differential diagnosis of a:
      i. *Periapical abscess.*
      ii. *Periapical cyst.*
      iii. *Periapical granuloma.*
      iv. *Periapical cholesteatoma.*
   c). The *radiopaque lesion* in the right maxillary sinus could be:
      i. *Periapical cemental dysplasia,* mature stage.
      ii. *Antrolith.*
      iii. *Osteoma.*
      iv. *Soft-tissue calcification* outside the sinus, such as a *calcified phlebolith.*

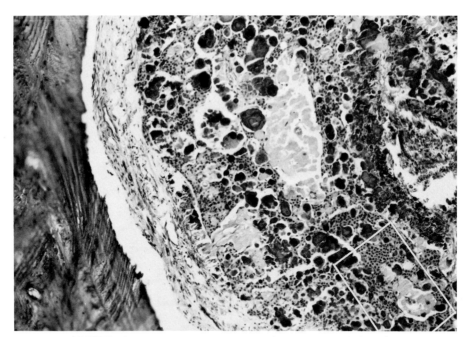

FIGURE 18B. Courtesy of Dr. R. C. Lachance, Montreal, Canada.

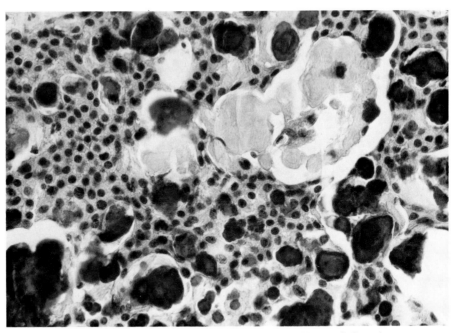

FIGURE 18C. Courtesy of Dr. R. C. Lachance, Montreal, Canada.

1. Differential diagnosis:
    a). *Calcifying epithelial odontogenic tumor (CEOT) of Pindborg.*
    b). *Central odontogenic fibroma.*
    c). *Keratinizing and calcifying odontogenic cyst (KCOC) of Gorlin.*

d). *Compound-complex odontoma.*
e). *Fibrous dysplasia.*
f). *Paget's disease.*
g). *Hyperparathyroidism.*
h). *Osteogenic sarcoma.*
i). *Chondrosarcoma.*

2. The diagnosis was a *Pindborg tumor (CEOT).*

Comment. Note that this lesion is often associated with an impacted tooth and is usually located in the posterior body of the mandible. Radiographically, the lesion often resembles "driven snow." Note that the histologic features of this lesion are classic.

CASE 19

If you said *chronic focal sclerosing osteomyelitis,* you get an "A" for effort. Note, however, the extensive destruction of the anterior ascending ramus.

In radiograph 19A, there is a notable finding: Usually a long-standing impaction has little or no visible follicular sac space or periodontal membrane space, and often the tooth appears ankylosed and even partially resorbed. In this case, a visible follicular space associated with drainage should arouse suspicion. With resorption of the ridge and trauma from the partial denture, an infection of the follicular space area would be an excellent working diagnosis. There is, however, one other finding: A follicular cyst was developing. Remember that folliciuar cysts or their incomplete removal may give rise to an ameloblastoma, a central epidermoid carcinoma, or a mucoepidermoid carcinoma. One now has these entities to consider in a differential diagnosis, as well as the chronic focal sclerosing osteomyelitis.

Upon biopsy this case was found to be a moderately well-differentiated *mucoepidermoid carcinoma.* The patient underwent a hemimandibulectomy and five years postoperatively no recurrence has been detected.

CASE 20

If you said mildly but positively *diabetic,* you would be correct. Most of the case history is typical for the unsuspected mild diabetic.

Comment. Remember that if you suspect the presence of diabetes and if the FBS level and findings on urinalysis are normal or high normal, the glucose tolerance test should be your next step.

POSTSCRIPT

The patient was treated with an oral hypoglycemic agent, and as her systemic problem became more controlled, the oral problem cleared up. The patient was successfully treated with osseous recontouring, several extractions, and a full-arch splint.

CASE 21

1. *Chronic suppurative osteomyelitis with pathologic fracture of the mandible* — right side.
2. Treatment:
   After sequestrectomy had been performed, the mandible was immobilized for a period of six weeks by means of extra-oral skeletal pin fixation. The microorganisms were found to be sensitive to erythromycin, and the patient received the appropriate therapy. Healing occurred uneventfully.

Comment. When culture and sensitivity tests reveal that the organisms are sensitive to erythromycin, long-term erythromycin therapy should be initiated, and the patient should be placed under close observation until resolution and healing have occurred.

CASE 22

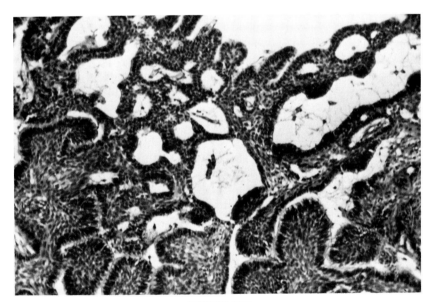

FIGURE 22*B*

Ameloblastoma (follicular type).

CASE 23

1. Differential diagnosis:
   a). *Globulomaxillary cyst.*
   b). *Periapical cyst, abscess, granuloma,* or *cholesteatoma.*
   c). *Periapical abscess associated with an odontogenic adenomatoid tumor.*

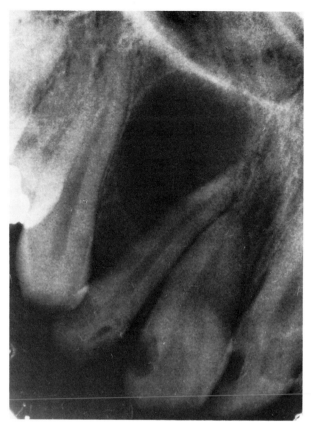

FIGURE 23D

Note. Although this lesion was not biopsied, the area resolved following the treatment that will be described shortly. A gutta-percha point inserted in the parulis and along the fistulous tract showed a continuity with the large radiolucency seen in the radiographs. This was probably a *periapical cyst* (note the thin radiolucent line circumscribing the distal two thirds of the area) that had become secondarily infected. Note, however, that based on radiographs alone, a *periapical abscess, granuloma, cyst,* or *cholesteatoma* cannot be definitively diagnosed, although this radiograph has the more typical appearance of a cyst. Also, one would not expect an abscess to cause displacement of the tooth. *Periapical granulomas* rarely exceed 1 cm in diameter and may be associated with root resorption. In a young patient who has a lesion in the maxillary anterior region, a diagnosis of *odontogenic adenomatoid tumor* should never be excluded. If the tooth was vital, the lesion would be typical of a *globulomaxillary cyst,* which is known to cause spreading of the roots of maxillary lateral and cuspid teeth.

2. *Root canal therapy; orthodontic realignment* and *retention;* and *post, core,* and *crown* the tooth.

CASE 24

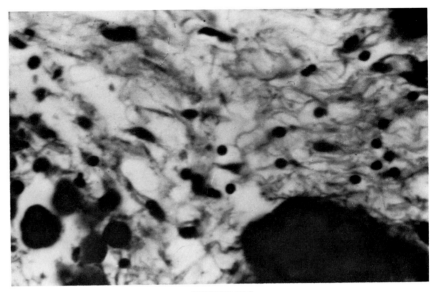

FIGURE 24C

The history, symptoms, radiographic findings, surgical findings, and biopsy report are typical of the *odontogenic myxoma,* which, indeed, this case was.

CASE 25

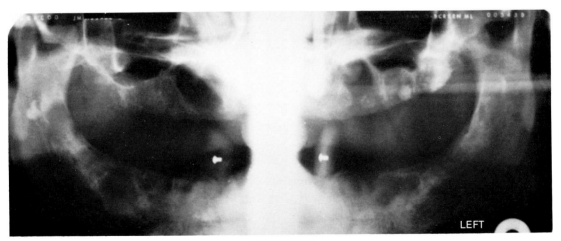

FIGURE 25B

If you said "a can of worms" or some such comment, you would be right. When faced with a radiograph such as this, one does not know what to think. Note the *large radiolucency in the mandibular right posterior region.* The area has a rough sclerotic border with several smaller, "punched-out" areas nearby. This area is certainly of concern. Note also the *large periapical radiolucency in the left mandible* as well as the *area in the left maxilla* that is expanding the floor of the maxillary sinus. There also appears to be some *sclerotic bone or "bone scar"* in the area. There are *numerous retained root tips,* and two of the three remaining teeth are *carious and peridontally involved.* A full-mouth clearance was performed, and material that was enucleated from the large area in the right mandible was submitted for pathologic examination. The report was consistent with "residual dentigerous cyst," and healing was uneventful. All the areas resolved, and the patient received his dentures just a short time before he retired.

CASE 26

This was a *periapical cyst,* and this lesion is included to demonstrate the difficulty in diagnosing large maxillary cysts occupying the entire maxillary antrum. Note that if a cystic sac was not present, the injected radiopaque material would have drained from the posterior opening of the maxillary sinus into the nasopharynx.

Note also that the lesion was "stomp positive," a term coined by Dr. Tom McDavid of Memphis, Tennessee. This finding should alert the clinician to the presence of increased intra-antral pressure.

CASE 27

"Jaw cyst–basal-cell nevus–bifid rib syndrome" (Gorlin-Goltz syndrome).

Note. The jaw cysts are keratocysts, as can be seen in the photomicrograph. In viewing the radiograph, note the large size of the cyst in the left mandible (arrow a) as well as the tremendous displacement of the 12-year molar tooth bud in the right mandible caused by that keratocyst (arrow b). There is another large keratocyst in the left maxilla. Examples of bifid ribs may be seen in areas c, d, and e of Figure 27E.

CASE 28

If you said *follicular* or *dentigerous cyst* associated with the impacted mandibular left third molar, you would be correct.

Note, however, that the following features should have alerted you to the fact that this was a *follicular keratocyst:*

1. Unusually large size.
2. Scalloped borders.
3. Resorption of associated root apices.
4. Delineation by a well-defined, thin radiopaque border, especially in the superior portion.

Comment. It is important to follow these patients closely postoperatively, as keratocysts tend to recur, usually within three to five years.

CASE 29

Fibrous healing defect (apical scar).

CASE 30

1. *Traumatic cyst* (hemorrhagic cyst; solitary bone cyst).

Comment. Note how the area extends up between the teeth and roots in a "smooth, undulating" manner. Note also the associated loss of the lamina dura. Although expansion occurs with some frequency, root resorption and/or displacement of the teeth are relatively infrequent findings. This lesion may occur without a history of trauma.

CASE 31

If you said *odontogenic keratocyst,* probably *primordial type,* you were quite correct, as the biopsy proved in this case.

Comment. Note the following common features of odontogenic keratocysts: large size and lobulated borders, mimicking the ameloblastoma and other similar lesions; and the clinical finding of white, "curdy" material, which is the desquamated, keratinized layer of the epithelial lining, which also contributes to the "cloudy" appearance of the area in the radiograph. Note that the outline of the soft-tissue swelling can be seen radiographically.

CASE 32

If you said *monostotic fibrous dysplasia,* you were indeed correct.

Note the ground-glass appearance of the bone in the Waters' view as well as the extent of the sinus involvement. The lack of subperiosteal erosion was an important clue in ruling out hyperparathyroidism, in which this is almost always seen.

When fibrous dysplasia is diagnosed in a patient of this age, Albright's syndrome should be ruled out by examining for the following: other bony lesions; café au lait spots; precocious puberty and other endocrinopathies.

CASE 33

1. The two main problems are:
    a). *Osteoarthritis* in the *left* TMJ due to:
        i. Trauma five years ago.
        ii. Long-standing myofascial pain dysfunction (MPD) syndrome.

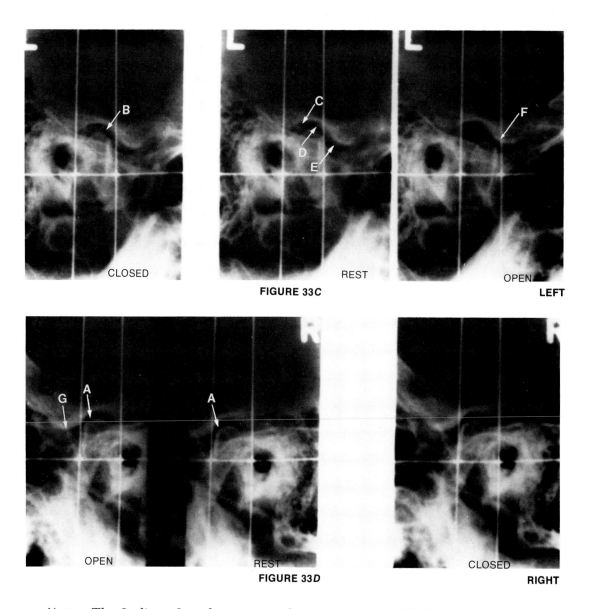

FIGURE 33C   LEFT

FIGURE 33D   RIGHT

Note. The finding of tenderness to palpation in the *left* TMJ is an indication of an inflammatory problem and is not usually a finding in MPD syndrome.

Note. Although psoriasis is an inflammatory dermatologic condition associated with accelerated cell turnover time, it may also affect certain joints, and there are several reported cases of psoriatic involvement of the TMJ.

    b). *Myofascial pain dysfunction syndrome* (TMJ dysfunction syndrome; Costen's syndrome).

Note. The remainder of the history and physical findings are diagnostic of a coexisting MPD syndrome. In fact, a subacute MPD syndrome probably existed prior to five years ago, and the blow to the TMJ precipitated the onset of symptoms. Other traumatic episodes, such as a lengthy dental appointment, a night of excessive bruxism, or a day of severe clenching, have been known to precipitate the onset of symptoms. In this case, either the trauma to the *left* TMJ five years ago or the long-standing MPD syndrome could be responsible for the osteoarthritis seen now.

Note. The presence of osteoarthritis alone cannot adequately explain the tender muscles and headaches.

    2.   Radiographic evidence of pathology:
        a). *Right* TMJ – slight flattening of the anterior head of the condyle; the cortical bone remains intact (arrow A).
            Left TMJ — distinct flattening of the anterior head of the condyle; the cortical layer of bone is lost (arrow B).
            Left TMJ — inflammation of the mucosal lining, as can be seen by the slight opacity between the head of the condyle and the posterior portion of the glenoid fossa (arrow C), the anterior portion of the glenoid fossa (arrow D), and the articular eminence (arrow E).
        b). *Radiographic evidence of deviation:* In the *left* TMJ, the head of the condyle moves anteriorly to the articular eminence (arrow F) in the open position; whereas in the *right* TMJ, the condyle does not move at all in the open position (arrow G). This radiographic finding confirms the clinical finding of deviation.

    3. *Physical finding relating to clicking:* The symptom of clicking is usually related to a lack of coordination between the superior and inferior heads of the external (lateral) pterygoid muscle on the affected side, and usually one or the other is in spasm, as confirmed by the finding of tenderness on palpation.

    4. *Treatment:*
        a). Salicylates and other anti-inflammatory drugs used for arthritis, such as ibuprofen.
        b). Treatment of the MPD syndrome is in three phases:
            i. Acute — analgesics and muscle relaxants to relieve the muscle spasm.
            ii. Exercises or myotherapy to relax the muscles that are responsible for the acute symptoms.
            iii. Exercises or physiotherapy to retrain the patient to use her jaw properly.

Note. In at least one study by Dr. George Zarb, it has been shown that once phase three has been completed, patients who have their occlusion equilibrated will not have recurring symptomatology as frequently as those whose occlusion is not equilibrated.

Note. During the three phases of treatment, one must also aim to correct the parafunctional habit, such as bruxism, clenching, or gum chewing. In addition, the practitioner must establish rapport with the patient, using supportive psychotherapy throughout. This will help to bring out the emotional factors involved, and once recognized, these must ultimately be managed if recurrence is to be avoided.

Note. There are many other approaches to therapy, all of which seem to meet with success in individual practitioners' hands. This is one of the interesting features of this self-limiting condition.

5. *Factors for monitoring progress:*
   a). Pain: decrease or absence.
   b). Decreased or absent muscle tenderness.
   c). Regression of TMJ noises.
   d). Greater maximum opening, especially beyond 40 mm.
   e). Greater freedom of movement, with decrease or absence of pain.
   f). Eradication of parafunctional habits.
   g). Recognition by the patient of the coexistence of emotional problems and evidence that the patient is taking steps to reduce them.

CASE 34

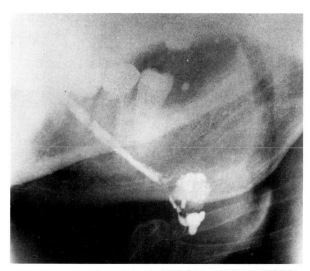

FIGURE 34*B*. Injection phase 2–5 ml.

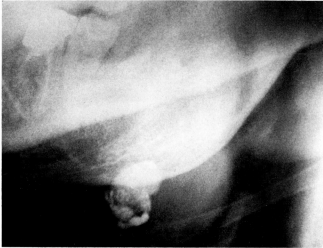

FIGURE 34*C*. 30-minute emptying. Delayed emptying time.

Left submandibular gland — sialolith. Note that the sialogram is helpful in establishing the presence of a salivary calculus as opposed to a calcified lymph node; an osteoma of the mandible, sclerotic bone, or calcified soft tissue, such as is seen in some scars.

Treatment consisted of removal of the left submandibular gland.

1. Further questions:
    a). *Do you get headaches?*
    b). *If so, where?*
    c). *Do you get "stuffed-up"?*
    d). *Do you experience postnasal drip, especially at night or upon awakening?*

2. Further examinations:
    a). *Palpation of the maxillary sinus* bilaterally in the area of the canine fossae.
    b). *Transillumination* of the maxillary sinus.
    c). *Waters' sinus radiographic view.*

3. Impression: *Maxillary sinusitis.*

Note. The history of odontalgia, which is difficult to localize in the maxillary teeth, may be the only symptom of maxillary sinusitis. Sensitivity to percussion and "stomp positive" odontalgia are also clues, as are negative pulpal and periodontal findings.

Note. In this radiograph, both maxillary sinuses are "cloudy" — an important clue in the diagnosis. This may represent a fluid level and/or the inflamed, thickened mucosal lining of the sinus. Waters' sinus view is helpful, as are the lateral and posteroanterior views.

4. *Antibiotics and antihistamines.*

CASE 36

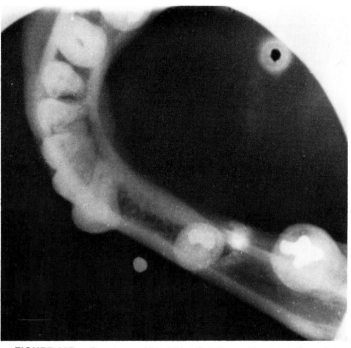

FIGURE 36B. Courtesy of Dr. Elliot Goldberg, Montreal, Canada.

The radiograph that should be taken is the *occlusal view* as seen here (Fig. 36–B). Note that the pellet is buccal to the ridge.

CASE 37

1. Mesial and distal *caries* in the left mandibular second molar (tooth number 37).

    2. Differential diagnosis:
        a). *Central ossifying fibroma of bone. Central cementifying fibroma of bone.*
        b). *Benign cementoblastoma.*
        c). *Calcifying epithelial odontogenic tumor of Pindborg.*
        d). *Fibrous dysplasia.*
        e). *Focal sclerosing osteomyelitis.*
        f). *Gigantiform cementoma.*

    3. *The most likely choices are a and b.* Note, however, that the benign cementoblastoma often obliterates the outline of the root of the involved tooth. The central cementifying or ossifying fibroma of bone grows slowly in all directions, and as it becomes more calcified, the radiographic appearance of the lesion becomes a large, round radiopaque mass that is well delineated from the surrounding bone, as can be seen in this case. The Pindborg tumor, fibrous dysplasia, and focal sclerosing osteomyelitis may not have such distinct borders, and none of them have the same tendency to grow equally in all directions. The gigantiform cementoma is a rare condition.

    This case proved to be a central cementifying fibroma of bone.

CASE 38

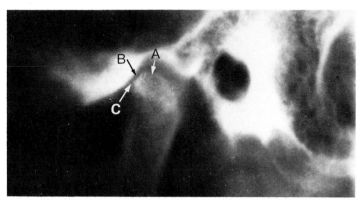

FIGURE 38F

1. In the closed position, the pertinent tomograms show that both condyles are placed anteriorly in the fossa, that is, there is an *anterior loss of joint space.* According to Wainberg, the condyles should be located centrally in the fossa.

The left condyle appears normal. The right condylar head shows a loss of the bony cortex in the anterior area (arrow A) as well as a flat table-like area (arrow B) and the beginning of spur formation (arrow C). All of these are early *arthritic changes*.

    2.   *Myofascial pain dysfunction syndrome.*

    3.   *Initially, treatment is similar to that outlined in case 33.* However, the anterior open bite is a problem. The referring dentist provided records showing that when a crown was made two years ago, the patient's occlusion was normal. In this case, *a balanced, wedge-shaped occlusal splint* was constructed, and eventually several *third molars were extracted.* This gave her more occlusion anteriorly, but the anterior open bite remained. Nonetheless, wearing the modified occlusal splint keeps the patient asymptomatic.

CASE 39

    1.   Differential diagnosis for epulis-like growth on the gingiva:
       a). *Peripheral giant cell granuloma.*
       b). *Peripheral odontogenic fibroma.*
       c). *Pyogenic granuloma.*
       d). *Peripheral Gorlin cyst.*
       e). *Epulis fissuratum (denture hyperplasia).*
       f). *Carcinoma.*

    2.   This was a *gingival carcinoma with erosion of the underlying bone.*

Comment.   Note that in edentulous areas, all of these lesions may have originally been central in bone. Shafer states that in edentulous areas the peripheral giant cell granuloma shows a pathognomonic peripheral "cuffing" of the bone.

CASE 40

Cherubism.

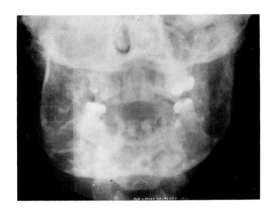

FIGURE 40*B*

CASE 41

As can be seen in the transorbital view of the right temporomandibular joint, the entire *head of the condyle has been fractured* off and appears to be united at the neck of the condyle. The free end of the neck of the condyle has now become the articular surface of the mandible, thus producing the facial asymmetry of this patient.

CASE 42

Traumatic cyst (hemorrhagic bone cyst, static bone cyst).

CASE 43

1. *Mesiodens.*

2. Figure 43A: *Standard maxillary occlusal view.*
   Figure 43B: *Maxillary crossfire view.*

3. Figure 43A: The *advantage* is the excellent view of the shape and size of the lesion.
   The *disadvantage* is that the mesiodens cannot be definitively located buccally or lingually.
   Figure 43B: The *advantage* is the excellent method of locating the lesion palatally or labially.
   The *disadvantage* is the poor view of the shape and size of the lesion and the much longer exposure of the patient to radiation.

CASE 44

1. Differential diagnosis:
   a). *Chronic diffuse sclerosing osteomyelitis secondary to previously existing periodontal disease.*
   b). *Multiple periapical cemental dysplasia* (cementomas).
   c). *Fibro-osseous disease of bone,* such as Paget's disease or fibrous dysplasia.

2. Although biopsy can help rule out the fibro-osseous disease of bone, it is more difficult to rule out the first two conditions, as they may represent variants of the same condition. Note the small "ball-like" opacities in the right and left maxillae, which strongly resemble cementomas. The large, sclerotic areas in the mandible, along with a fistula and impending sequestration, are typical of diffuse sclerosing osteomyelitis. Both of these conditions have a predilection for black, middle-aged females. Recently, the use of the gallium scan has greatly aided diagnosing chronic osteomyelitis in a definitive manner.

CASE 45

Bilateral fracture-dislocation of the mandibular condyles.

CASE 46

1. *Oro-antral fistula.*

2. An oro-antral fistula is treated by *excision of the fistulous tract and closure of the communication* between antrum and mouth. A variety of surgical techniques have been described, such as a palatal pedicle flap, a Berger sliding flap, a gold plate, and others.

    Before attempting closure of an oro-antral fistula, it is imperative that the involved sinus be completely free of all infection and that when the communication is closed, there is good drainage from the antrum into the nose. The patient's general physical condition must be evaluated, and any underlying systemic condition (e.g., diabetes) must be treated prior to closure.

CASE 47

1. *Static electricity* (arrow A).
2. *Static electricity* (arrow B).
3. *Static electricity* (arrow C).
4. *Developer artifact* (arrow D).
5. *Chin-rest shadow* (arrow E).
6. *Left ala of the nose* (arrow F). We apologize if we fooled you on this one.

CASE 48

POSTSCRIPT

Yes. Tomography of the left temporomandibular joint area is indicated. *A tomogram revealed a fracture of the mandibular neck.* This was treated conservatively by prescribing a soft diet and exercises.

CASE 49

Ameloblastoma.

CASE 50

Lingual mandibular salivary gland depression.

Note. In case 50B, the condition is bilateral.

CASE 51

Bilateral—mucous retention phenomenon of the maxillary sinus.

CASE 52

1. *Partial anodontia.*

2. *Hereditary anhidrotic ectodermal dysplasia* and *therapeutic radiation at an early age.*

CASE 53

1. *Numerous small, punched-out radiolucent areas,* the borders of which appear smooth and regular, are seen in the skull, the mandible, and the vertebrae. The lesions vary in size but range from 4 to 7 mm.
2. Diagnostic impression: *Multiple myeloma.*

CASE 54

1. There is a *radiopaque mass* arising from the floor and medial wall of the left frontal sinus. There are varying degrees of radiopacity. The borders appear smooth and regular.
2. Microscopic examination of the lesion revealed an *osteoma,* and indeed this is the most common location of this lesion.

CASE 55

Paget's disease of bone (osteitis deformans).

Although not pathognomonic for the condition, this x-ray picture is typical of Paget's disease. The overall radiographic picture is one of diffuse areas of osteoporosis and osteosclerosis that give a "cotton wool" appearance. The cortices of bone may be thickened; the jaws become enlarged, in particular the alveolar processes; and teeth may show root resorption or hypercementosis. The history of this case is also typical. A helpful laboratory finding is very high levels of serum alkaline phosphatase.

CASE 56

Impression: *Osteopetrosis, malignant recessive type* (marble bone disease).

Comment. Note that this condition is characterized by normal bone deposition but a lack of resorption, ultimately choking out the bone marrow spaces. Even though the liver and spleen become enlarged as they attempt to compensate for the decreased bone marrow function, the patient ultimately becomes anemic, and death is usually the result of the anemia or an associated infection. Radiographs are very helpful in the diagnosis, and the generalized opacity of all the bones is diagnostic of osteopetrosis. Note, however, that this must be distinguished from a condition characterized by an increased thickness and density of the cortical bone known as generalized cortical hyperostosis (van Buchem's syndrome) and from Pyle's disease (metaphyseal dysplasia) and craniometaphyseal dysplasia.

CASE 57

Impression: *Eagle's syndrome* (elongated styloid process neuralgia, styloid syndrome).

Note. Depending on the author or the study, a styloid process in excess of 2.5 cm to 3.0 cm in length is considered elongated. Note also that although the styloid process may be elongated bilaterally, not all patients experience bilateral pain, and indeed not all patients with elongated styloid processes become symptomatic.

One theory on the development of this condition is that the scarring that results from tonsillectomy causes increased tension on the stylopharyngeal ligament. This ultimately produces an elongated styloid process that irritates the ninth cranial nerve, thus producing pain. There are several other theories as to the pathogenesis of this condition as well.

One may palpate the elongated styloid process from the tonsillar fossa, and the treatment is simply to surgically reduce the length of the elongated process.

CASE 58

1. Differential diagnosis for the *2-cm radiopaque lesion in the left maxillary sinus:*
    a). *Osteoma,* arising from the medial or lateral wall of the maxillary sinus.
    b). *Juvenile nasopharyngeal angiofibroma.*

    Note. This lesion arises in the nasopharynx and usually causes anterior bulging of the posterior wall of the maxillary sinus.

    c). *Mucous retention phenomenon* of the maxillary sinus.

FINAL DIAGNOSIS: This case proved to be an *osteoma.*

CASE 59

1. Abnormalities:
    a). *Radiation stunting* of the permanent teeth in the right maxilla and of the posterior permanent teeth in the right mandible.

b). *Radiation stunting* of the maxillary incisors and the first bicuspid on the contralateral side.

c). *Failure of development* of many permanent teeth on the right side and of the maxillary second bicuspid on the contralateral side.

d). *Incomplete development of the mandible* on the right side, especially in the angle area, producing facial asymmetry. It is for this reason that the rib was transplanted.

Note. The remaining teeth in the affected areas should be preserved and infections, trauma, and surgery should be avoided if possible owing to the ever-present possibility of the patient developing osteoradionecrosis.

CASE 60

You have seen this before. Try to recall the possibilities for multilocular radiolucent lesions.

1. Differential diagnosis:
    a). *Ameloblastoma.*
    b). *Pindborg tumor (calcifying epithelial odontogenic tumor of Pindborg).*
    c). *Aneurysmal bone cyst.*
    d). *Central giant cell granuloma.*
    e). *Odontogenic myxoma.*

2. This case proved to be an *ameloblastoma.*

Note. In the lateral tomographic view (Fig. 60B), the soft-tissue swelling may be readily seen and represents a perforation of the lesion at the crest of the ridge. Note that in the panoramic view, which is in effect a tomogram or laminogram, the crestal bone appears intact. The lateral jaw tomographic series was carried out in order to determine if any portion of the lesion had perforated the mandibular canal. This is necessary for determining the surgical procedure required.

CASE 61

1. Differential diagnosis:
    a). *Hyperparathyroidism* (primary or secondary).
    b). *Paget's disease of bone.*
    c). *Fibrous dysplasia.*

2. Definitive diagnosis: *fibrous dysplasia* (see Table 1.)
The proof of diagnosis was by *biopsy* (see Table 1.)

TABLE 1. DEFINITIVE DIAGNOSIS OF FIBROUS DYSPLASIA

Differential Diagnosis	Radiographic Findings				Laboratory Tests				Biopsy		
	Cotton-Wool Bone	Ground-Glass Bone	Loss of Lamina Dura	Radiolucent and/or Radiopaque	Elevated Serum Calcium	Elevated Urine Calcium	Elevated BUN	Elevated Alkaline Phosphatase	Presence of Giant Cells	Presence of Fibrous Connective Tissue and Bone Trabeculae	Mosaic Bone Reversal Lines
Primary hyperparathyroidism		X	X	X	X			X	X		
Secondary hyperparathyroidism		X	X	X		X	X if renal disease is present	X	X		
Paget's disease of bone	X	X	X	X				X			X
Fibrous dysplasia		X	X	X				X		X	

137

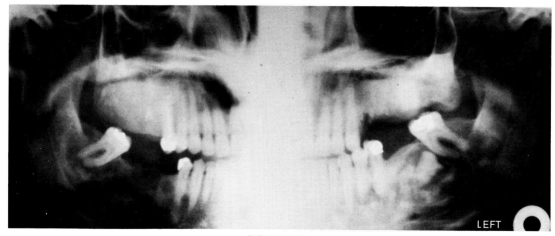

FIGURE 61B

Note. This condition may be characterized by radiopaque areas, radiolucent areas, or both. This case demonstrates all three of these possibilities:

1. Radiopaque areas — maxilla, right and left.

2. Radiolucent areas — mandible, right.

3. Mixed — mandible, left.

CASE 62

1. The 15-minute emptying film clearly demonstrates a filling defect in the hilus of the left parotid gland. Retention of the dye occurs proximal to this area, while the main duct shows minimal emptying. There also appear to be several other radiolucent areas in the secondary duct proximal to the blockage. Comparison of this film with the terminal opacification film shows some emptying of the gland but at a markedly reduced rate. Normal emptying time is approximately 10 minutes.

2. *Mucous plug(s)*, left parotid gland.

CASE 63

1. Differential diagnosis:
   a. *Odontoma.*
   b. *Adenomatoid odontogenic tumor (AOT) (adenoameloblastoma).*
   c. *Pindborg tumor (CEOT).*
   d. *Ameloblastic odontoma.*

FINAL DIAGNOSIS: This lesion was treated by excisional biopsy and proved to be a *compound composite odontoma.* Note that on panoramic films, smaller lesions are rather indistinct in appearance, and these films should be supplemented by intra-oral periapical views.

Comment. Note that the AOT frequently occurs in young females, has a propensity for the maxillary anterior region, and is often associated with an impacted or unerupted tooth. Unlike the ameloblastoma, the ameloblastic odontoma occurs in young people, and it is for this reason that all odontomas should be submitted for histopathologic examination. Although odontomas may recur, the ameloblastic type has a greater propensity for recurrence, and because of its locally destructive nature, it requires very careful and regular radiographic follow-up. The Pindborg tumor, like the ameloblastoma, tends to occur in adults over the age of 35 years; however, it may occur in young people and is often associated with an impacted, unerupted tooth.

CASE 64

In this radiograph, the following abnormalities should be noted:

1. *Follicular cyst* associated with an unerupted supernumerary maxillary fourth molar. The cyst occupies the entire left maxillary tuberosity.

2. *Mesially impacted supernumerary maxillary fourth molar* or third molar. An adequate history would determine if the third molar had been extracted.

3. *Distal pseudohyperostosis.* This small, bony bulge may be noted distal to both mandibular second molars. These areas sometimes become traumatized, causing the patient to complain of pain in the area. These small, bony bulges are normal variants and should not be mistaken for frank pathosis.

CASE 65

There is evidence of extensive *pneumatization* of the maxillary sinuses. The floor of the sinus extends well down the mesial root surface of both maxillary first molars as well as into most of both maxillary tuberosities.

The large radiolucent area at the right angle of the mandible below the mandibular canal is compatible with a radiographic diagnosis of *lingual mandibular salivary gland depression.*

There is a *fracture of the right coronoid process.* This is the probable source of the patient's complaint.

In the maxillary anterior area under the pontic, there appears to be a fibrous healing defect or a focal osteoporotic bone marrow defect of the jaws or a prominent incisive foramen.

In the apical third of the root of the left central incisor there appears to be a residual infection associated with a lateral canal or a prominent superior foramen of the incisive canal.

At the apex of the mandibular central incisors, the radiopaque area is compatible with the genial tubercles.

CASE 66

1. Note the impacted left mandibular third molar associated with resorption of the distal root of the second molar.

2. With this in mind you should have the following in your differential diagnosis:

    a). *Fibrous healing defect.*

    b). *Focal osteoporotic bone marrow defect of the jaw.*

    c). *Residual cyst, granuloma, infection.*

A biopsy would establish a definitive diagnosis, which in this case was the *fibrous healing defect.*

Note. The fibrous healing defect is thought to develop when there is a loss of the buccal and lingual cortical plates and their periosteum. The periosteum is thought to be the source of mesenchymal cells having the osteoblastic potential necessary to form the new bone.

CASE 67

The findings consist of a *congenitally missing permanent second bicuspid* and a large *follicular cyst.* The follicular cyst is associated with a horizontally impacted second molar. The cyst appears to have posteriorly displaced the developing third molar, which has not yet begun to calcify.

Confirm by biopsy of the cystic area.

Note. This lesion was indeed a follicular cyst, and once this was enucleated, the second molar erupted in a normal manner. Also note that prior to calcification, the developing tooth buds resemble a well-delineated radiolucency. These should be recognized for obvious reasons. If, however, a developing tooth bud is submitted for histopathologic examination, it is important to inform the pathologist, as the young, developing papilla may be indistinguishable from the odontogenic myxoma.

CASE 68

1. In the right mandible, there is a *developing supernumerary bicuspid tooth* with incomplete root formation associated with divergence of the roots of the first and second bicuspids.

In the left mandible, there is a large *radiopaque area* that measures 2.5 cm × 2.5 cm, consisting of several tooth-like masses and possibly one impacted supernumerary bicuspid. The distal superior aspect of this area is surrounded by a 4-mm radiolucent area. This lesion is associated with divergence of the roots of the first and second bicuspids.

2. Impression:

a). *Right mandible,* developing supernumerary bicuspid.

b). *Left mandible,* compound composite odontoma associated with an impacted supernumerary bicuspid and a follicular cyst.

Confirm by biopsy.

Comment. Note the elongated styloid process on the left side.

CASE 69

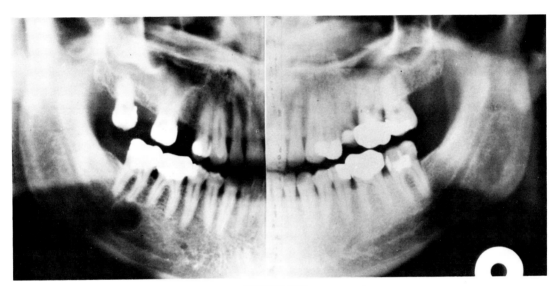

FIGURE 69*B*

1. The lower right second molar (tooth number 47) has a large restoration, possibly a full crown with deficient mesial and distal margins. There is an additional buccal or lingual restoration below the gingival margin of the large restoration.

Intimately associated with the apex of the mesial root of this tooth is a circular, radiolucent area that measures 1.2 cm in diameter and that is well delineated by a distinct sclerotic border. The inferior border of this lesion is intimately associated with and appears to be encroaching upon the superior portion of the mandibular canal.

2. Differential diagnosis:

a). *Periapical cyst.*

b). *Periapical granuloma.*

c). *Periapical abscess.*

d). *Periapical cholesteatoma.*

Note. Biopsy proved this lesion to be a *periapical cyst.*

1. Extraction of the teeth should be considered in cases involving any one of the following:
    a). Poor oral hygiene and/or poor patient motivation for future good oral hygiene.
    b). Advanced periodontal disease.
    c). Advanced caries and/or pulpitis and its sequelae.

Extraction of teeth should be considered especially when
    a). A major portion of the major and/or minor salivary glands is within the portal of radiation.
    b). A major portion of the supporting bone, especially the mandible, is within the field of irradiation.

In this case a full-mouth clearance with alveolectomy was recommended prior to radiotherapy.

2. *In the area of the sigmoid notch of the right mandible*, including the coronoid process and the superior portion of the anterior border of the ramus, there appears to be some erosion, possibly due to invasion by the carcinoma in the right tonsillar fossa. There also appears to be destruction of the right maxillary tuberosity, mimicking advanced periodontal disease.

These findings were confirmed by other radiographic studies, and a combined surgical and radiotherapeutic approach was used.

CASE 71

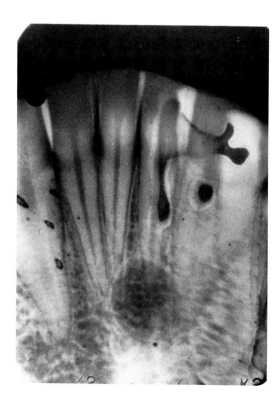

FIGURE 71*B*

1. The lesion is at the *apex of the mandibular left central incisor.*

Comment. Note the periapical film of this area, which is highly suggestive of a cyst.

2. Differential diagnosis:
   a). *Anterior lingual salivary gland depression.*
   b). Central, unilocular, benign lesion such as *hemangioma.*
   c). *Periapical cemental dysplasia,* osteolytic stage.
   d). *Periapical cyst, granuloma, abscess,* or *cholesteatoma.*
   e). Developing *odontoma* or *ameloblastoma.*

3. No. In this case, the positive response to the electric pulp test is confusing, but this sometimes occurs in a nonvital tooth and may result from conductivity by fluids in the pulp canal or an anticipatory response by the patient or a second vital pulp canal in the same tooth. Also, note that the lesion is indistinct on the panoramic film, which may be due to the fact that the area is located just outside the focal trough of the machine used. Suspicious areas should be examined further with intra-oral, periapical, or other views.

In this case, surgical exploration was carried out, and the area was found to contain purulent material and what appeared to be some epithelium. On histologic examination, the lesion was found to be a *periapical granuloma,* once again showing that periapical lesions with sclerotic borders may not necessarily be cysts and that those lesions smaller than 1 cm in diameter may very well be periapical granulomas.

4. *Developer artifact.*

CASE 72

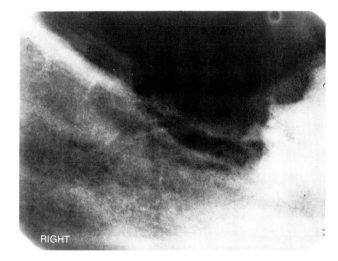

FIGURE 72B

1. *Osteoradionecrosis.*

2. Three factors are usually required for this condition to develop, although radiation alone can be the etiologic factor.

a). *Radiation* (therapeutic).
b). *Trauma.*
c). *Infection.*

3. The following precautions are helpful in preventing osteoradionecrosis when surgery is being contemplated.

    a). Adequate history and enquiry concerning the *anatomic location of the portals used.*

    b). If the prognosis is reasonable, *exhaust other methods of treatment before surgery.* Example: endodontics versus extraction.

    c). Protect the patient with *antibiotics* before, during, and well after the procedure.

    d). If the case involves an extraction, *an atraumatic procedure* should be performed if possible; effect primary closure.

    e). *Continue antibiotics and follow-up.*

4. Sequestration may continue, and resection of the jaw may be necessary.

CASE 73

The sialogram shows a typical "ball in hand" picture in the lateral ramus view, which is typical of a space-occupying lesion in the inferior portion of the superficial lobe of the parotid gland. This "ballooning" effect is caused by displacement of secondary and smaller ductules by the lesion. In the anteroposterior view, however, the discontinuity of some third- and fourth-order ductules is an "ominous" sign, suggesting a possible malignancy.

POSTSCRIPT

This lesion proved to be a *pleomorphic adenoma* (benign mixed tumor).

Comment. Note that this is the most common type of benign salivary gland neoplasm, and though the lesion is usually encapsulated, tumor cells are often found within the connective tissue capsule, thus accounting for possible recurrence of this lesion.

CASE 74

1. *Complex composite odontoma.*

2. *Ameloblastic odontoma;* it is for this reason that all odontomas, no matter how obvious radiographically, should be biopsied. Although both of the above conditions may recur, the ameloblastic variety has a much greater frequency of recurrence and thus requires a vigilant follow-up. Recurrence indicates the necessity for a more radical surgical procedure.

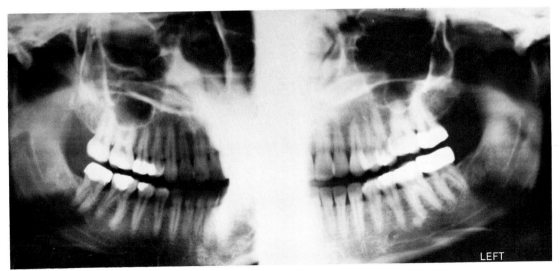

FIGURE 75*B*

Now that you have seen the second radiograph, it is obvious. This turned out to be a clip on the side of the neck of a turtleneck ski sweater.

Note. In viewing these two radiographs, the astute radiologist should not fail to report the small *radiopaque area at the apex of the mesial root of the mandibular left first molar*, which could be:

1. *Osteosclerosis (bone scar)*.
2. *Focal sclerosing osteomyelitis* (secondary to pulpal inflammation associated with the deep restoration).
3. *Exostosis* or *osteoma*.
4. *Sialolith* (within Wharton's duct).
5. *Calcified soft tissue* such as a phlebolith, scar, or lymph node.

With the foregoing in mind, the following further procedures are recommended:

1. Occlusal view.
2. Possibly a sialogram.
3. Pulp tests (heat, cold, and electric).
4. Soft-tissue film of the cheek.

CASE 76

1. A 1.5-cm radiolucency, occupying the midportion of the left body of the mandible, extends mesially to the lateral incisor and distally to the second premolar. The area has a faint "honeycomb" or "soap bubble" appearance. Associated with this radiolucency is

anterior displacement of the developing cuspid to the central incisor region and posterior displacement of the developing first bicuspid to the mesial region of the first molar. The area is oval-shaped and well delineated by a thin cortical outline. There is no evidence of expansion in this view. Immediately superior to this lesion, at the crest of the alveolar ridge, is a 5-mm area of sclerotic bone, possibly a sequela of a previously infected deciduous tooth.

    2.   Differential diagnosis:
        a).   *Central giant cell granuloma.*
        b).   *Aneurysmal bone cyst.*
        c).   *Ameloblastic fibroma.*
        d).   *Odontogenic myxoma.*
        e).   *Central hemangioma.*
        f).   *Primordial cyst of a supernumerary tooth.*
        g).   *Ameloblastoma.*

    3.   This lesion proved to be a *central giant cell granuloma*, and this is a typical example of this lesion.

Choices b, c, and d would have all been excellent, since all three lesions could occur in identical circumstances. Choices e, f, and g are also very possible but more remotely so.

CASE 77

    1.   The deciduous teeth were decalcified and were submitted for histologic examination. Both radiographs and histologic findings were compatible with a diagnosis of a rare condition known as *enamel and dentin aplasia.* The large pulp chambers resemble the changes seen in *hypophosphatasia.*

    2.   Radiographically, the permanent teeth in the maxillary right quadrant are typical *"ghost teeth,"* otherwise known as regional odontodysplasia. These teeth were not submitted for histologic examination for the presence of the characteristic interglobular dentin with the irregular, gnarled pattern of dentinal tubules.

    3.   This probably represents a case of *focal dermal hypoplasia,* otherwise known as the Goltz syndrome. Holden, J. D., and Ackers, W. A.: Amer. J. Dis. Child, *114*:292, 1967.

CASE 78

    1.   *Nondisplaced fracture, right body of the mandible.*

    2.   Differential diagnosis:
        a).   *Phleboliths.*
        b).   *Multiple parotid salivary stones.*
        c).   *Calcified scar tissue.*
        d).   *Foreign body fragments.*
        e).   *Artifact (projected from an item of clothing).*

    Comment.   Note the horizontal opaque strokes seen on the *left* side originating from these objects on the *right* side.

3. Arrows A through N:
   A). *Chemical artifact* (developer).
   B). *Metal pin or chin positioner.*
   C). *Dorsum of the tongue.*
   D). *Mental foramen.*
   E). *Malar process of the zygomatic arch.*
   F). *Articular eminence.*
   G). *Sigmoid notch.*
   H). *Coronoid process.*
   I). *Mylohyoid line.*
   J). *Ball of gauze.*
   K). *Floor of maxillary sinus.*
   L). *Mandibular canal.*
   M). *Maxillary tuberosity.*
   N). *Right mandibular condyle.*

CASE 79

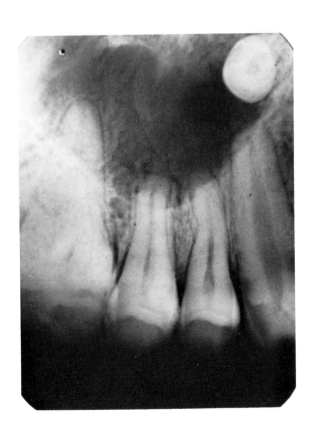

FIGURE 79B

1. Differential diagnosis:
   a). *Follicular cyst associated with an impacted supernumerary tooth.*
   b). *Follicular cyst associated with a developing odontoma.*
   c). *Osteoma,* arising from the anterior wall of the maxillary sinus.
   d). *Antrolith.*

2. Comparing the right and left sinus spaces, one can see that on the left side, the sinus is much higher up. Additionally, the radiolucent area appears to be intimately related to the radiopaque object. The radiopaque object resembles a mesiodens or a supernumerary cuspid tooth. The roots of the right maxillary cuspid and bicuspids are shorter than on the left and appear to have been resorbed. The horizontal radiopaque shadow present in the panoramic film but absent in the periapical film represents the dorsum of the tongue and should not be mistaken for a fluid level or a soft-tissue space-occupying lesion.

This was a *follicular cyst associated with a supernumerary tooth,* as shown on biopsy.

CASE 80

Persistent jaw pain with an associated paresthesia is an ominous sign of serious disease. This patient was found to have *metastatic disease* in the left mandible from a primary carcinoma in the left lung. Note that the metastatic lesion in the mandible was what caused the patient to seek treatment and that odontalgia is often a presenting symptom. Had the panoramic film not been taken, the lesion might not have been discovered. Since the discovery of Batson's plexus, metastatic disease to the jaws is easily explained.

Comment. Note that the lesion consists of a 1-cm radiolucency in the third molar area, which has infiltrated a large portion of the ramus with destruction of the anterior border.

CASE 81

1. *Periodontosis.*

Comment. Note that periodontosis is of unknown etiology. It commonly affects black female juveniles and typically affects the areas described here in the early and intermediate stages of the disease.

2. Note that within ten months of transplantation, there is almost complete regeneration of the lost alveolar bone. In the anterior region, however, the conservative approach to therapy failed, and both lateral incisors were subsequently lost.

3. Comparing Figure 81C with Figures 81A and 81B, note the following changes in the transplanted teeth:
   a). *Some root formation* has occurred and still remains incomplete four years postoperatively.
   b). *The pulp chambers have been completely obliterated.* This is often seen in transplanted teeth.
   c). Note the plane of occlusion in Figure 81B. All of the transplanted molars were placed well below the plane of occlusion. Note in Figure 81C that *the transplanted molars have erupted into occlusion.*
   d). Note the *stunted root formation.*

e). In the lower molars especially, note the *"fat-man girth"* appearance of the roots relative to the crown. The periodontal ligament space is outside the "bulge," suggesting an unusual clinical impression of *hypercementosis*, presumably a response to increase the attachment area to make up for the deficient root length.

CASE 82

Cleidocranial dysostosis (Cleidocranial dysplasia).

CASE 83

1. *It is possible.* If a patient develops a postextraction osteitis or "dry socket," the condition is extremely painful and may persist over a period of several months if not properly treated. Note, however, that in this three-week postoperative film, there is no evidence of bony sequestra nor does the surrounding bone have a mottled appearance, which would suggest an osteomyelitis. The periapical area, in fact, appears to be resolving.

2. The important radiographic finding is the *complete destruction of the left maxillary tuberosity* in both the periapical and panoramic views. This was originally overlooked. Surgical exploration of the maxillary buccal vestibule revealed a rather reddish, fungating mass adjacent to the left maxillary tuberosity.

POSTSCRIPT

Biopsy revealed *malignant melanoma.*

CASE 84

1. In the case of the *mandibular left first molar,* there is an *altered mesial interproximal contact area* due to the crowding of the left second bicuspid. This has resulted in the development of a deep pocket between these two teeth. Note that the *bifurcation involvement* in the mandibular left first molar is radiographically more severe than the bifurcation involvement of the mandibular right first molar, and the presence of the deep mesial pocket on the left side has certainly contributed to the greater destruction on that side.

In the case of the *mandibular left third molar,* there is a *mesial loss of periodontal support.* This developed as a sequela of the extraction of the mandibular second molar and the resultant mesial tipping of the mandibular left third molar. The mesial "pseudo pocket" that developed contributed to the present degree of periodontal disease. Note that radiographically, there appears to be a *bifurcation involvement* in the mandibular left third molar as opposed to no bifurcation involvement of the mandibular third molar on the right side.

Comment. Note that radiographically, there are deep pockets between the maxillary first and second molars on both sides.

2. Apart from the obvious answer stressing *home care* and *routine recall examinations*, the following could have helped to prevent the more severe periodontal destruction in the mandibular left quadrant:

 a). *Reestablished proper contact* between the second bicuspid and the first molar by orthodontics or *extraction* of the second bicuspid and prosthetic reconstruction.
 b). *Replace the extracted second molar* by prosthetic reconstruction; or to have attempted to "save" the second molar in the first place.

CASE 85

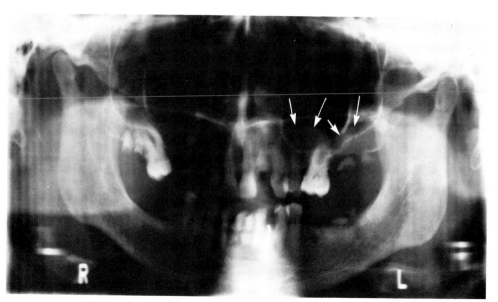

FIGURE 85C. Courtesy of Dr. Olaf Langland, San Antonio, Texas.

1. In Figure A, there is a pronounced *mucositis* of the lining mucosa, involving especially the posterior half of the mucosal lining. In the anterior half, a more pronounced *mucous retention phenomenon* appears to be developing and may be a sequela of the former condition. Both of these conditions may develop as a result of very early acute periapical inflammation or chronic periapical or periodontal disease. Notably, both of these conditions are also seen in the absence of periapical or periodontal inflammation. In figure B there is a large mucous retention cyst occupying much of the left maxillary sinus.

CASE 86

1. The unerupted maxillary right third molar is *partially re-sorbed* in a manner that resembles a "ghost tooth" (regional odontodysplasia) – a condition whose histologic features differ from those of a resorbed tooth.

Comment. Note that resorption is often associated with impacted or unerupted teeth of long standing. The resorption may affect not only the involved tooth but also portions of erupted teeth in close proximity to the involved tooth.

CASE 87

1. *Acute pericoronitis* associated with the mandibular left third molar. Note the *crescent-shaped radiolucent area* associated with the distal portion of the crown of the mandibular left third molar. Radiographically, this is highly suggestive of pericoronitis. Note that on the right side there is radiographic evidence of pericoronitis, which in this case is subclinical but may be responsible for the tender lymph node on that side.

2. *Congenitally missing mandibular second bicuspids.* Note the "submerged" deciduous second molars.

CASE 88

1. *Recurrent odontogenic keratocyst, follicular (dentigerous) cyst type.* Note the relatively large size of the area and the "cloudy" appearance of the cyst.

TOOTH NUMBERING CHART

Midline Maxilla

Right

18	17	16	15	14	13	12	11	21	22	23	24	25	26	27	28
Third molar	Second molar	First molar	Second bicuspid	First bicuspid	Cuspid	Lateral	Central	Central	Lateral	Cuspid	First bicuspid	Second bicuspid	First molar	Second molar	Third molar
48	47	46	45	44	43	42	41	31	32	33	34	35	36	37	38
Third molar	Second molar	First molar	Second bicuspid	First bicuspid	Cuspid	Lateral	Central	Central	Lateral	Cuspid	First bicuspid	Second bicuspid	First molar	Second molar	Third molar

Left

Mandible Midline

INDEX

Numbers in italics refer to illustrations. Numbers followed by t refer to tables.